CATFLEXING

This book is dedicated to my husband Jonathan.
Without your constant love and support,
Catflexing would still be my secret pastime.

CATFLEXING

A Catlover's Guide to Weightlifting, Aerobics & Stretching

Stephanie Jackson

Photography by John Werner

TEN SPEED PRESS
Berkeley, California

The exercises and nutritional information contained in this book are generally safe and effective. However, despite every effort to offer expert advice, it is not possible for this book to predict an individual person's or cat's reaction to a particular exercise or nutritional program. The reader should consult a qualified physician and veterinarian. Neither the publisher, Ten Speed Press, nor the author, Stephanie Jackson, accept responsibility for any effects that may arise from attempting the exercises or following the nutritional advice in this book. No animals were harmed to make this book.

1☉

Ten Speed Press
P. O. Box 7123
Berkeley, California 94707

Excerpts from *The Complete and Up-to-Date Fat Book* © 1993 by Karen Bellerson. Reprinted by persmission of Avery Publishing Group, Garden City Park, NY.

A Kirsty Melville Book

Design by Catherine Jacobes

Photography by John Werner

Cover photo by Jonathan Snyder

Library of Congress Cataloging-in-Publication Data
Jackson, Stephanie.
Catflexing / by Stephanie Jackson.
    p.   cm.
        ISBN 0-89815-940-7
1. Cats--Exercise. 2. Aerobic exercises. 3. Cats. I. Title.
            SF446.7.J335   1997
        613.7'1--dc21   97-19407
                        CIP

Printed in the United States
First Printing, 1997
1 2 3 4 5 - 01 00 99 98 97

❖ CONTENTS ❖

ACKNOWLEDGEMENTS

TO BAD, WHOSE FEARLESSNESS is a constant source of inspiration and whose trust goes beyond words. Without your playfulness and fiery spirit, we would have never thought of Catflexing. And to Masi and Cochise, who have often taken a back seat to the "show kitty," you are both stars to me.

To Alicia and Lew, who supported me in more ways imaginable and who believed in this project sometimes more than I did. I love you both.

To John Werner, my photographer, who is the most patient man I ever met and by far the most talented. I thank you even more for your extreme sensitivity towards animals and for honoring Bad and Masi's feelings during the photo shoot.

To John Painter, my agent, who had enough faith for the two of us and who never doubted the potential of this project.

To Kirsty Melville for believing in Catflexing, Nancy Austin and Catherine Jacobes for their artistic direction, and special thanks to Kathryn Bear, my editor who has sheperded me through this process with the greatest of ease. It was also a thrill to hear her finally exclaim, "Good, Bad!"

To my mother, I love you dearly. Your long-distance phone calls to cheer me on really mean the world to me.

To the clan on the east coast: Brigette, Jon, Emily, Sam, Kathy, Greg, Evanne, Lauren, Jimmy, John, Debbie, Maxx, Sam, Janeann, Stan, Alicia, Brooke, and all my friends, your encouragement was always appreciated.

And to Taboo, who was once an excellent Catflexer.

INTRODUCTION

OKAY, SO I'M NOT THE MOST CONVENTIONAL PERSON in the world. Family and friends tell me I'm weird. Even my own mother has told me this for as long as I can remember. I couldn't help it if birds landed on my shoulder or tried to pull hair from my head to make their nests. I was an innocent bystander! To make me feel better, she'd tell me Webster's says that weird means unique. Well, that didn't make me feel any better! All I wanted was to be like my brothers and sisters, and what did unique mean anyway? As I've gotten older though, I've come to accept this "special" quality and I figure there's nothing wrong with being unique.

I was brought up in rural Pennsylvania, sandwiched between three older sisters and a younger brother and sister. My family was very active both indoors and out-doors. I remember spending endless hours as a child with the family gathered around the piano while my mother played our favorite songs. Some of us would sing, others would dance, and still others would do gymnastics. It was a three-ring circus. During the summer I spent most of my time in the woods hiking around inspecting every little creature possible. Animals soon became my best friends. Oddly enough, birds were naturally attracted to me; in fact, many animals have made strange appearances in my life including Bad, my cat, but you'll hear more about that later. You'd think I was related to Dr. Doolittle!

When I was growing up, my family had no choice but to protect my sensitiv-ity. I was an animal fanatic. They would walk on eggshells and fabricate elaborate stories every time my father left the house in his hunting clothes with his shotgun.

It got to a point that if he did bring anything home, he'd have to leave it at the neighbor's house. I used to interrogate the poor man, searching all of his pockets before letting him in the house. I had a fit the first time I saw a cowboy movie when the horses appeared to have been shot. And when Lassie injured his leg and was stranded without help, I held my breath for the entire episode. Television was never quite appealing after that. Perhaps it was that incident that solidified my purpose in life. I decided to be an animal rescuer!

Most little girls play with dolls and toys. I, on the other hand, ran a veterinary clinic out of my bedroom, which was full of injured animals that desperately needed my care. In my room I had birds, cats, dogs, squirrels, snakes, and bunnies. In my closet I had even more birds, cats, dogs, squirrels, snakes, and bunnies. Animals everywhere! Somehow word got around the neighborhood, and when animals were sick and needed to be taken care of, people would call me. Luckily, I had understanding parents. My tenacity and love were my animals' best medicine. I bandaged, splinted, stitched—you name it, I did it.

I have always been athletic. As a child, if I wasn't competing in a hand-walking contest, I was ice skating until my parents had to literally grab me and drag me off the ice. I took dance and swimming lessons, but my true love was diving. I was a cheerleader from seventh grade through my senior year. In spring and summer, I was a member of the track and softball teams, and in winter I was involved in gymnastics. I also loved golf and still do. During college, my main form of aerobic activity was biking and walking to and from class since I did not have a car. I also thoroughly enjoyed dancing and did that as frequently as possible.

After graduating from college, the reality of the working world hit. How was I ever going to get any exercise sitting at a desk? The thought of having to be one of those professional people racing to the gym after work was dreadful. But, as it turned out, that is exactly what I did. I lived in the gym for what seemed an eternity. And then I found my perfect exercise program.

Our Story

WHEN PEOPLE ASK HOW I conceived my Catflexing program I always tell them, "too many years spent at the gym." After years of working out in cold gyms, I decided that standing next to Mr. Amazon, who huffed and puffed, grunted and groaned, was not my idea of a good time. I was there to strengthen and tone, but the guys I generally shared the gym with were there to conquer and annihilate. The veins that popped out of their necks were bigger than my biceps. I often felt I had no business being there with my little 3- and 5-pound weights. Not only that, I wasn't having any fun. So I decided to go solo, get out of the gym, and do my workout program at home. Because of my many years of training, I felt I had more than enough discipline and knowledge to design a thorough program that would keep me interested. Little did I know my cats would be just as interested!

One day, as I was pumping iron with the music blaring, my cat Bad, in her very persistent way, wanted to be held. I didn't want to stop exercising, so I put down my weights, picked her up, and wrapped her little body around my shoulders. She didn't seem to mind the movement as I performed my lunges, so I did my usual three sets with her. The added weight of her eight pounds was perfect for this exercise, as I generally use weights that range

1

from three to five pounds each. So, I figured let's try another one. It was time for my bicep curls. I cradled the underside of her belly with both hands and began lifting her up toward my chest, then down, then up and down. I was sure she would leap out of my arms and run for the hills, but she totally trusted me and went with it. In fact, she began purring. I thought this was particularly strange, but thought to myself, we're onto something here. The true test was when I tried the behind-the-neck curls. This is a tough one to begin with, let alone with a cat. I positioned her safely above my head just as you would a barbell and pressed her up and down, up and down. She didn't flinch! I became curious, wondering if she had done this before, and with whom?! She was a pro! I continued with my entire set using Bad, and fascinated with our breakthrough. Needless to say, my dumbbells took a back seat, and Catflexing was born!

Bad and I did not have the most typical of meetings. In fact, Bad claimed me. I had no intention of getting a cat; the thought had never crossed my mind. One reason may have been that I lived in a condominium complex where pets were not allowed. Bad, however, must have thought she was the exception to this rule.

It was Christmas Day and as I was walking down the sidewalk beside my apartment, minding my own business, this young whippersnapper raced up the walkway and literally leaped into my arms. I've had many a cat in my day, and I tried to recall any of them doing that, but I couldn't think of one. Here I am, all dressed up ready to go to a holiday function, and I have a cat cradled in my arms. This ball of fur acted like we had known each other for eons, purring with content as I stood there holding her. I put her down and asked where she lived. She walked straight up to my doorstep as if she knew exactly what I had just asked and nonchalantly plopped herself down on my welcome mat. I knew I was in trouble. I told her to go home, and that I had to go, but thanks for the exuberant greeting, and have a wonderful Christmas.

Upon returning home from a day full of holiday cheer, I walked up the sidewalk and stairs to my apartment. Lo and behold, guess who was there? That's right. She greeted me with a purr and I went in to find her something to eat. After a quick nibble, she took off. For the next few weeks, she hung out at my doormat. I took her around the neighborhood, looking for her home. No one in the neighborhood knew a thing about her. I posted signs on her behalf 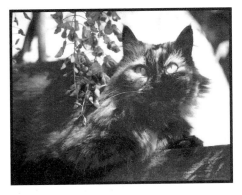 stating that she was lost and surely missed. I never received a call. It was during this initial bonding period that whenever I would see her I'd tell her in my goo-goo gaa-gaa voice that she was such a bad kitty. That was my way of telling her how much I adored her.

My newfound friend charmed me more and more every day. She would meet me at my car on my arrivals home from work. Like the genetic code that dictates eye color, she had one for distinguishing the sound of my car and running to greet me. She would sit at my front door for days on end, not crying to get in, but appearing relieved that she finally found her home. She would sleep on top of my car and welcome me to the day first thing in the morning, leaving behind her glorious little paw signature on my hood. No matter where I went, there she was.

One day, I was taking my garbage to the dumpster with my sidekick, of course, right beside me. My landlord came up to help me with my bags and walked with me to the bins. I was so nervous trying to think of ways to explain to this man that this was not my cat, although we did look like Mutt and Jeff. So—here I was walking with my landlord, making small talk, and pretending this furry little creature trotting between us didn't exist. He said, "I've noticed a cat around here the last few days. Is it yours?" I looked down at this little critter, and she looked up at me. I said, "No, I've never seen this cat

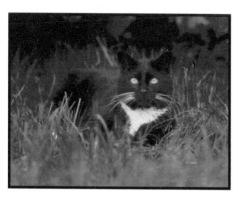

before." He said, "Okay," and we put the garbage in the dumpster. I turned and walked back toward my apartment—like clockwork, so did she. My landlord watched us from the walkway, and it was then I knew our days at this condominium were numbered.

I thought she was absolutely the kookiest cat I had ever met. I would open my door to allow her to come in for a visit, and she would spring from one piece of furniture to the next, never touching her feet to the floor. It was bizarre! Maybe she really did know I wasn't allowed to have pets. She would find her way into a cupboard, open it with her paw, and close it behind her. She still does this! She also had a thing for napping at other people's houses regardless of whether she knew them or not. I would be walking past a neighbor's apartment on my way home from an evening out, and I would see her through a window on top of someone's TV or curled up on the ledge of a windowsill. I'm not sure if the neighbors even knew she was there. I've lost count of the number of houses I've seen her in. She continued to do that for years. It used to make me so jealous when she'd come home with perfume scents on her fur, or a hint of smoke, like she'd spent the night in front of a fireplace! I've had neighbors whom I've never met leave notes on my door or call me and tell me that my cat slept in their beds and they had no idea how she got in. I'll never forget the time when my sister took me home from work one day, and as we were nearing my house, she noticed that in my neighbor's second story window there appeared to be a cat just like mine. I looked up, and sure enough, it was Bad on the inside looking out, sleeping on the ledge of someone's window. I knocked on the neighbor's door and told them my cat was in their house. They looked at me with a strange expression and denied it. I asked for permission to come in, and proceeded to show them.

It was a hopeless case. I finally realized we were destined to be together. She, of course, had known it all along. Well, as you may have guessed, I lost my apartment, along with a large deposit. However, I received the best Christmas present ever. I had called this little kitty "bad" for so long while helping her find a home that when I finally thought of naming her, nothing else fit. My friends think it's a little weird, though, when they hear me say with all sincerity, "Good, Bad."

Bad and I had lived together for about six years when one day a colleague of mine who was moving to another state brought me the cutest little kitten as a going-away gift. If someone had asked me if I wanted another kitty, I would have said no, emphatically. Bad was more than a handful. But when he put that six-week-old kitten in my hand, I turned to mush and the thought of this precious one going to someone else killed me. He told me that behind their farmhouse they had about fifteen feral cats and about eight of them had kittens. Before they moved, they wanted to find homes for the kittens. After thirty-odd cats had been rounded up and taken to an animal shelter, this little one came out from hiding, looking for his mother and for food. The rest is history.

I didn't want another adjective for a name, life with Bad was confusing enough. So, I named him Masi after a sleek Italian racing bicycle. Bad was not at all happy; in fact, I thought she would kill Masi. After all, Bad was a cat who thought nothing of chasing and attacking my neighbor's German shepherd, biting at his ankles during his retreat. We're talking seriously territorial. I would catch Bad clenching little Masi in her teeth and flinging him against the wall like a toy. After being scolded numerous times, Bad decided that if Masi wasn't going to leave, she would. She threatened our relationship by running away for days at a time, and under no circumstances would she come into the house. I was devastated. When she did come in the house, she made no attempt to even try tolerating the situation. My happy family fantasy was nothing but tension and chaos in reality.

I, Miss Psychology, decided intervention was necessary. My thoughts were consumed with how to achieve the desired result: Two cats romping together, living happily ever after. I tried everything under the sun to facilitate a truce. I referenced every cat book I could get my hands on. I called a few animal behaviorists and a couple of veterinarians for advice. I even called a psychologist. I spoke to everyone as if I had a rare disease and a cure had to be found immediately. I tried every remedy offered, but to no avail. Discouraged, I considered giving Masi up for adoption. Finally, at a party (ironically, at a veterinarian's home), the answer came to me. The vet told me I was trying too hard to facilitate something that they had to work out. Bad was probably more upset with the energy in the house than she was with the newcomer. It seemed too simple, but I had to give it a shot. He told me that when I stopped worrying, they would have the freedom to come to a solution by themselves. I tried it and I saw immediate results. Although some resentment remains, they have established a relationship that works for them. I've learned a lot from this lesson and have come to accept the imperfections that come with a family.

I don't see my Catflexing routine as weird, but rather an extension of myself and the connection I have with my two cats. I've been Catflexing with

Bad since she was a kitten, which means we've been working out together for almost nine years. Masi and I have been Catflexing for about three years. Frankly, I don't think he likes it as much as Bad. I hope in time he'll learn to love the sport, but I'll have to see. God only knows he needs to lose a few pounds. In fact, he's downright fat, but he really comes in handy during my chest set when I want to use heavier weights.

Most of our days are like clockwork. Bad and Masi always wait for my return home from work, which is usually about 5:30 PM. When Bad hears my car, she runs into the street and waits like a valet to greet me. I live in a rural area with little traffic, so it's okay. She'll often jump right into my car in full purr when I open the door. Masi, who is a bit more conservative, watches from a safe distance at the end of the walkway. This is one of our most special times, the "Mom is Home" ceremony! Together, we all walk up the narrow winding sidewalk with Masi dropping to roll for me at least twice. For those of you who have roll-happy kitties, you know how charming this can be. Bad generally leaps onto the deck railing to get even closer to me and to keep a close watch over Masi's antics. She then scurries up the tree adjacent to my house to get a better view, I suppose, but who really knows? In 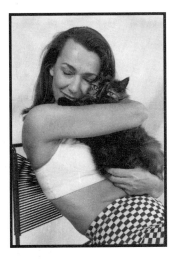 the meantime, I praise Masi for his generous rolls. Bad lets out a selfish hiss, displaying her insecurity with the attention given to Masi. For the big finish, I rattle my keys. Bad leaps down from her tree, and we all go inside together.

As I unwind from my day and prepare for working out, Bad and Masi snack on some crunchy dried cat food. They watch as I change into my workout clothes and put on my motivational music, which consists of disco music and other hard-driving beats. This is a dead giveaway that we will definitely be Catflexing tonight. By now they can hardly contain themselves; they intertwine their little bodies between my legs, rubbing on my ankles and purring. It's such a tease to them because they know they have to wait for me to return from my daily run. Sometimes Bad follows me down the street, meowing the entire way as if to say, "I want to come for a run with you." When this happens, I always stop running and take her for a walk. I realize she needs her aerobic activity as much as I do, plus, it's a great bonding session. We will walk only as far as the street's end, then turn around and sprint home together. My neighbors often do a double take, and sometimes they stop me and say, "Do you know you are walking your cat?" I look down at Bad and say, "Yes, I know." What's the big deal about walking a cat? After we get back home, I praise her and tell her to stay, then continue with my run.

Upon returning from my run, I change the music to their favorite band, The Pet Shop Boys, and our Catflexing begins. Our workout generally lasts about 30 to 45 minutes, depending, of course, on how Bad and Masi are feeling. Immediately following our workout, we always stretch for a good 15 to 20 minutes.

THE COMPETITION BEGINS

I think some people are born with natural athletic abilities. I also believe some people are born with higher competitive spirits than others. I was born with both. Fortunately, or unfortunately (I haven't figured this out yet), I have always loved competition and the rush it gives me, no matter what the sport is.

After about five years of Catflexing with Bad, I was getting very good at it, and I decided I wanted to share it with other people. I wanted to get together with a circle of friends to work out. I also wanted the camaraderie and opportunity to share cat stories because, believe me, there are many when you undertake a program like this. But how was I going to involve others with my obscure pastime? What would people think when they hear I work out with my pets?

I scratched my head on this one for about a month. Should I advertise in the paper? Should I recruit from health clubs? Skywriting is too expensive, so that was out. So was a commercial spot during Oprah. Then it came to me. I decided to go to all of the local pet stores, the really big ones that always have some type of marketing hype, and ask the managers if I could do an exhibition, a Catflexing exhibition. Some of the looks and responses I got were as if I had just asked if I could torch the store with their family tied up in back. I remember one man almost running away after I asked him. I think I heard him muttering something about 911 as he turned on his heel and fled. He probably though I had just escaped from Bellevue. I didn't take the rejections personally because I knew it was just a matter of time before someone gave me a chance.

Finally, I found a little old pet store owner who was so intrigued by my Catflexing proposal that he wanted me to do an exhibition immediately. A vendor had canceled at the last minute, so I had a spot on Saturday...three days away! I prepared my introduction speech and recruited a few friends for a quick critique. They patronized me politely, feeding me the familiar "Oh, Steph, you're so silly," when deep down I knew they thought I had stepped off the edge. Nonetheless, they supported me and gave their critiques. I put up posters in the pet store and the store owner mentioned the upcoming event to his patrons. Needless to say, I was nervous. Would they laugh at me, like my friends and family did?

Saturday arrived, my big debut, and I was amazed at the crowd of people that showed up. I think most people were there to see a circus sideshow.

Catflexing? Then what? An elephant on a pogo stick? A little section of the store was cleared out and I sat in the front on a tall stool addressing the crowd. Bad sat on another stool right beside me in her carrying case. I wondered how she was coping with this; after all, this was her first public appearance as well. From what I could gather, she was pretty indifferent. In fact, she was doing better than I was.

I began my talk on the overall benefits of nutrition and exercise for both cats and owners. My speech was very well received in that the question and answer period lasted for an entire half-hour. People were genuinely interested. I realized I had better get to my demonstration, as I was only scheduled for one hour. It was going so well!

Right before I took Bad out of her case, a million scenarios raced through my mind. Would she freak out with all these strange, new faces? Would she panic and jump up on one of the twelve-foot-high cat food can displays, or freeze and act is if she'd never Catflexed before? I didn't know which would be more embarrassing. I ordered myself to stop the self-torture. I was working myself into a frenzy that I didn't want Bad to sense. I opened the cage and lifted Bad out to introduce her to the public.

Everyone ooohed and aahed. Of course, I could have pulled out a tarantula and they would have responded the same way; after all, these were animal lovers—my favorite kind of people. Bad surprised me. She was a total ham. She was a stage actress, working the crowd, poised and ready to be flexed. She knew exactly why we were there and what we had to do. We had an outstanding Catflexing demonstration for an appreciative audience. People actually applauded. Who ever would have thought?

It was after this exhibition that my phone started ringing with requests for information on Catflexing. Catflexing was catching on like wildfire! More pet stores invited me to demonstrate. People started calling me "Dr. Catson, the Cat Lady." I got letters from catlovers wanting my advice not only on Catflexing, but everything under the sun relating to their cats. I even got an invitation from the manager who initially thought I was nuts. The small demonstrations evolved into regular group sessions and, ultimately, local competitions were arranged. The rest is history.

Now that you know the history, I'll let you in on what the judges are looking for in a Catflexing competition. Most of you will be Catflexing for the sole purpose of working out, but for those fitness buffs with that competitive spirit, it's always handy to know you can go to the top with your cats.

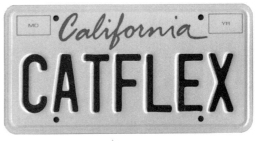

The competition consists of three categories. The first is judging the overall shape and definition of your body. The judges evaluate you from head to toe, giving you a rating from 1 to 10 on each body part; your score is derived from averaging that total.

The second category consists of rating the individual five-minute routine. This routine is judged on its overall composition, which is done to music. The judges are looking for proper technique, difficulty, mistakes, showmanship, musical interpretation, and chemistry between cat and owner. An overall score is then tallied.

Last, but not least, a score is given to your cat. Each cat is inspected from head to tail. The judges look for overall appearance, definition, and disposition. (I've seen a few judges get bitten by contestants. Needless to say, these cats and their owners were *not* the winners.) An average between all three categories is calculated and whoever has the most points wins.

Before You Start

IN THIS BOOK I'M GOING TO SHOW YOU how to use a Catflexing program step-by-step. The program is designed to give you shape and muscle definition. Many women have asked me if Catflexing will give them those big and bulky muscles bodybuilders get. I reassure them that my program will not do that. A definition workout consists of using lighter weights and higher repetitions. There is not enough weight with even the heaviest cat to build bulk.

Catflexing may feel foreign at first, but with practice, it gets easier. All you need to begin this program is motivation, patience, and the obvious, a cat.

MOTIVATION

Motivation is the key to everything. We all would have the bodies of professional athletes if we had their motivation. But I'm not asking for eight hours of sweat a day. All I'm asking is that you simply pick up your cat for approximately 20 minutes a day. If you own a cat, you may already do this, in which case, all you need to do is hold your cat a little differently than normal. This is where the motivation comes in. You will feel awkward, and guaranteed, so will your cat. But this awkward feeling will diminish as you continue. You may not be successful during your first few attempts. In fact, you may never be successful with certain cats. Nonetheless, give it your best until you are certain that you don't have the right workout partner.

PATIENCE

Because working out is not innate to cats, your patience is essential. It is important that you try to make this as fun as possible for your cat. If you have a special way of talking to your cat, now is the time to do it. If you feel anxious, so will your cat. It is very important to keep your cool and appear to know what you're doing. Your cat will pick up on your energy and trust this new activity.

A couple of weeks before beginning your program, I suggest holding your cat in various positions so it won't be startled. The more you handle your cat in different positions, the easier Catflexing becomes. Praise your cat after each handling so it feels rewarded for being handled and looks forward to the next session. It takes patience to get over this hump, but I'm sure you can do it.

THE CAT

Now for the obvious: The cat. If you do not have a cat, see about borrowing your neighbor's. Even if you do have a cat, sometimes borrowing your neighbor's cat isn't such a bad idea because your pet will not always be in the mood to work out. We all know how even-tempered our precious little ones are, now don't we? Are you ready? Put on those gym shorts and let's get started!

NINE CONSIDERATIONS BEFORE CATFLEXING

1. Exercise slows the aging process, for people and for animals. I've been Catflexing with my cat Bad for nine years now and though she's a cranky old ball of fur she has the bones of a teenager. Be very gentle if you are going to use an older cat for your Catflexing program. Remember, each cat year equals five to seven human years. I don't know about you, but if I were sixty or seventy years old, I wouldn't want someone flipping me around in unthinkable ways! Older cats are prone to arthritis which limits their flexibility, thus making it difficult to perform the positions needed. I would not recommend starting a Catflexing program with a cat older than eight years old.

2. Before you undertake a Catflexing program, see your physician for an exercise stress test and a physical evaluation. If this is the first time you are attempting a workout program, it is imperative you get a clean bill of health before starting. If you are an active person who frequently works out, then it is not as critical, but it's always a good idea to have a yearly physical regardless of how often you exercise.

3. Periodic medical check-ups are just as important for our feline friends. Although it may seem that you are the only one exercising since you are the one lifting, your cat gets her share of exercise by tensing certain muscle groups in an effort to maintain balance during the routine.

4. Water, water, water! You can never get enough! How much water should you drink? The recommended amount is seven to eight glasses a day. If you work out, increase the number of glasses to at least twelve. And always be sure to put out a fresh bowl of water daily for your beloved workout partner.

5. Emphasize safety and proper technique at all times. Although cats generally land on their feet, don't assume this will be true all of the time. It is possible to injure yourself and your cat if you do not perform the exercises correctly. In this book I provide detailed directions on how to handle your cat and how to execute each exercise. In addition to safety, this ensures that you are training the proper muscles. Please follow the directions carefully.

6. Catflexing is only one part of achieving overall health. Always warm up before an exercise program and stretch at the end of it. You will prevent injury to your body and keep it supple.

7. Rest is equally as important as training. Working out regularly is great, but overdoing it can be hazardous. Taking time off is essential for the body to recover and help prevent injury. Besides, cats like to nap much of the time and you wouldn't want to disrupt that, would you?

8. Always start an exercise program slowly. Many people get overly ambitious in the beginning and we all know what happens then—we get very sore, or we injure ourselves. It takes at least six months for our bodies to adjust to an exercise program working out three times a week. So keep it simple in the beginning. Both you and your workout partner will be glad you did.

9. Keep in mind that you will not see immediate results. Give yourself at least a couple of weeks of regular Catflexing, and before long, you'll see some incredible physical changes, you'll feel different about yourself, and your relationship with your cat will be better than ever.

The Exercises

THERE ARE THREE COMPONENTS of a complete workout: Aerobics, toning, and stretching. Catflexing falls into the toning category, although aerobics is part of the overall program.

BICEPS

Standing Catbell Curls

Stand with your knees slightly bent and your pelvis slightly tucked forward. With your arms extended, hold your cat with a palms-up grip. Keep your elbows close to your rib cage and don't let them move backward or forward. Slowly curl your cat up to your chest, then lower it down to a full extension. Inhale as you raise your cat, and exhale as you lower it. I recommend 3 sets of 10 to 15 repetitions, depending, of course, on your cat's tolerance. Do this exercise slowly and methodically; otherwise, the less trained cat may become nauseous.

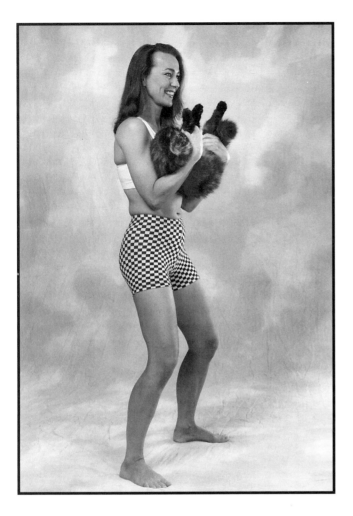

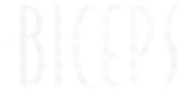

BICEPS

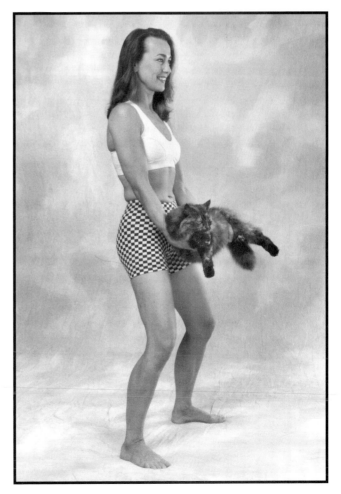

TRICEPS

Tricep Cat Extension

Stand with your knees slightly bent and your pelvis gently tucked forward. Don't arch your back. Hold your cat gently but firmly under its shoulder blades and pelvis. Keeping your biceps as close to your head as possible, press your cat directly over your head. Try not to let your arms wobble. After a brief pause with arms extended straight, lower your cat behind your head as far as possible. Then, using the strength of your triceps, extend your cat back up to the straight-arm position. Breathe normally throughout the exercise. I recommend 3 sets of 10 to 15 repetitions. A little hint: Be patient with your cat; this is a hard one to master and is frequently their least favorite.

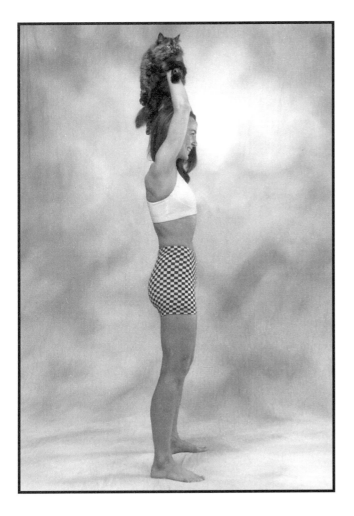

TRICEPS

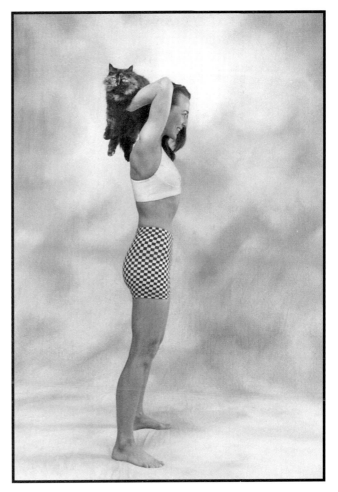

Cat Dips

Sit on the edge of a chair with your cat sitting across your lap. Slowly scoot out from the chair, allowing your hips to be suspended. Your feet should be securely planted on the ground (or on the balls of your feet, for advanced Catflexers). In this seated position, keeping your elbows tucked behind you, lower yourself to a reasonably comfortable position. Don't let your elbows flare out to the sides. Slowly push yourself back up to a full extension, without locking your elbows. I recommend 3 sets of 12 repetitions. For some odd reason, Bad sometimes likes to lie on her back during this exercise.

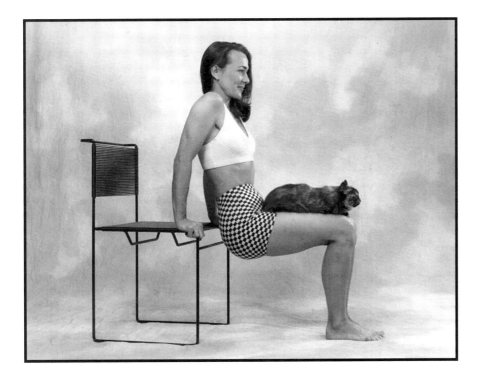

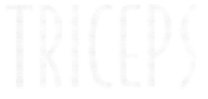

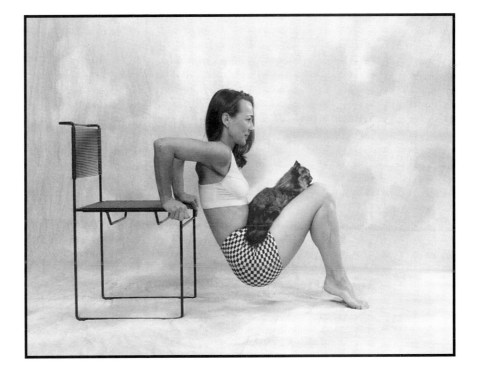

CHEST

Kitty Push-ups

There are two ways to do push-ups: On your knees (kitty-style) or on your toes (cat-style). For beginners, I recommend doing the push-ups in the knee position. I prefer this position. When doing push-ups from the knee position, keep in mind that the pivot point from the floor is the knees, and not the hip. Have your cat lay across your shoulders or back and go for it. I suggest 3 sets of 12 repetitions. See next page for Cat Push-ups.

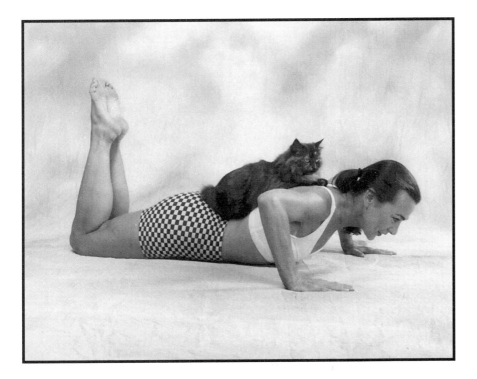

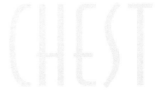

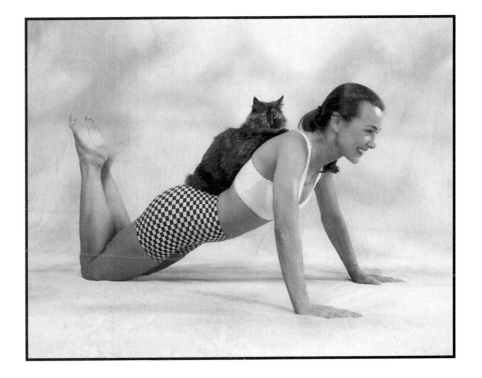

Cat Push-ups

For cat push-ups, start from a prone position with your palms on the floor at chest level, placed slightly wider than shoulder-width apart. Exhale as you push yourself up to a straight-arm position, keeping your back and legs straight. Inhale as you lower yourself to the point at which your chest barely touches the floor. This is an excellent exercise for toning the pectoral muscles of the chest, your triceps, and upper abdominal muscles. I recommend 3 sets of 12 repetitions. My tip for cats reluctant to stay on your back during this exercise: Put a few bite-size pieces of your cat's favorite snack on your upper back. It's guaranteed to do the trick!

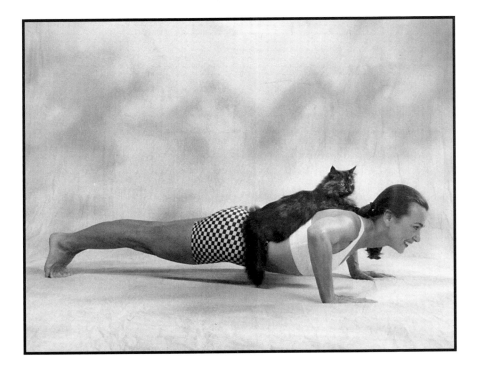

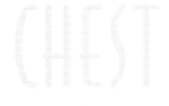

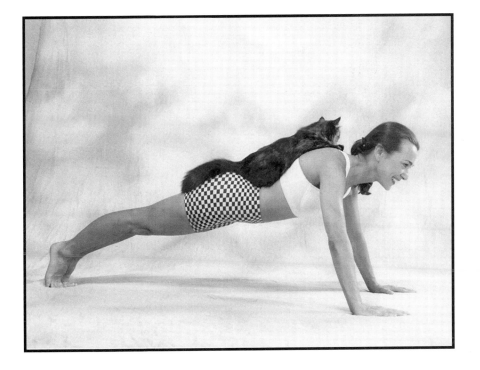

Catbell Press

Lie on your back, either on the floor or on an exercise bench. Position your cat comfortably across your upper chest. Firmly cradle the underside of your cat's belly. Exhale as you extend your arms vertically, inhale as you lower your cat. Always bend your elbows directly to each side for maximum stress to your pectoral muscles. I recommend 3 sets of 12 repetitions.

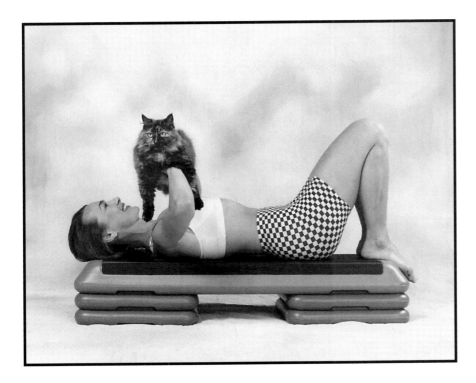

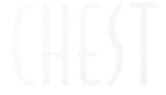

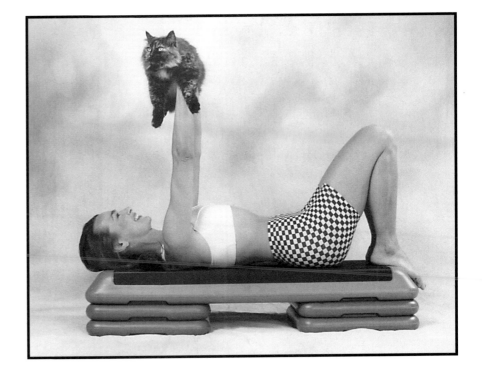

Cat Pullovers

Lie on your back with your knees bent and your arms fully extended directly behind your head. Hold your cat under its belly with your palms facing up. Exhale, and slowly raise your cat directly above your chest, keeping your arms straight. Pause, then inhale while slowly lowering your cat back to the floor. On an exercise bench, the pull is a bit more challenging. I recommend 3 sets of 13 repetitions.

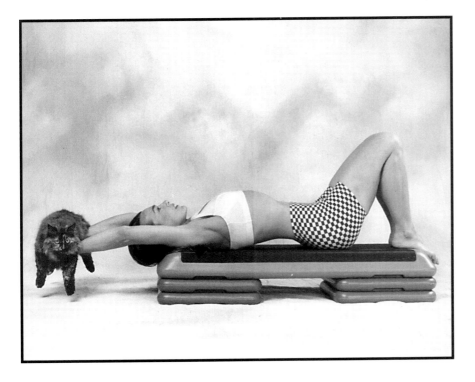

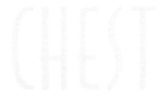

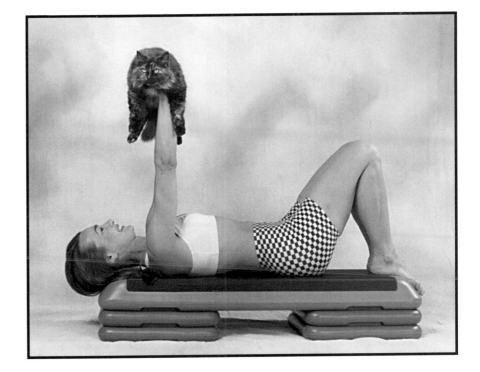

BACK

Upright Cat Row

Stand with your knees slightly bent and your pelvis gently tucked forward. Hold your cat with an overhand pronated grip on the underside of its belly. Try to grasp your cat behind the front legs and in front of the back legs for even weight distribution. Bad was perfect for this exercise because she is very small and I was able to get my hands around her waist. Pull your cat straight up, keeping it very close to your body, and raising your elbows toward the ceiling and slightly backward with your elbows. Exhale as you pull your cat up and inhale as you lower it. When your are holding your cat correctly, this is also a nice stretch for her.

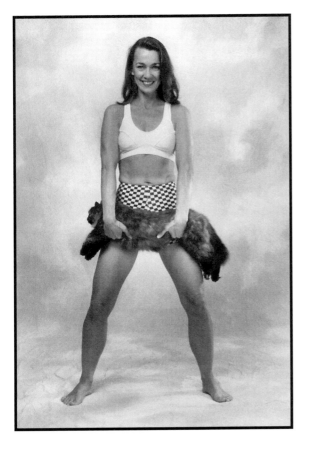

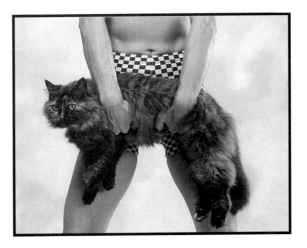

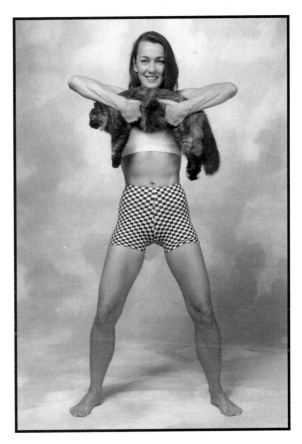

BACK

Cat Bows

Stand erect with your cat draped across your shoulders and your feet positioned slightly closer than shoulder-width apart. Keeping your legs straight and holding on to your workout partner, bend forward from the waist until your torso is almost parallel with the floor. Pause for a moment with your face forward and your back slightly arched. Slowly return to the starting position. Remember to tighten your stomach muscles and breathe normally. This exercise is particularly good for strengthening your upper back, which will help you maintain good posture. I recommend 2 sets of 10 to 12 repetitions.

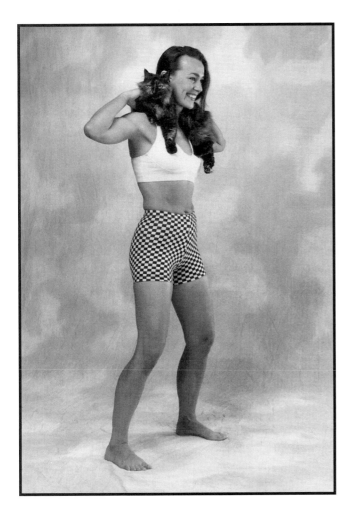

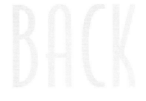

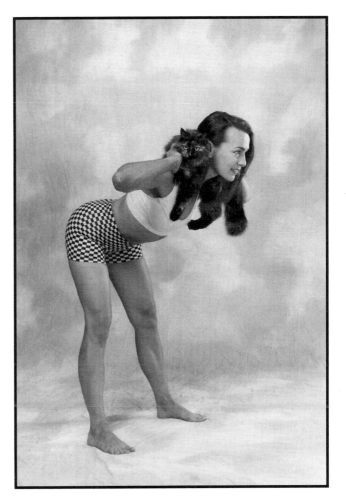

Dead Cat Lift

Position your cat directly in front of your feet. With your legs straight and your arms fully extended, bend and take hold of your cat behind the front legs and in front of the back legs. Slowly come to an upright position, pulling your shoulders slightly back. Pause for a moment, then slowly bend forward from the waist, keeping your legs straight and arms fully extended. When bending forward, go as far as you can toward the floor. This exercise is great for the lower back. However, if you have a heavy cat, be careful not to strain yourself when executing this exercise. If you experience any discomfort, either use a lighter cat, or skip this one. I recommend 2 sets of 12 repetitions.

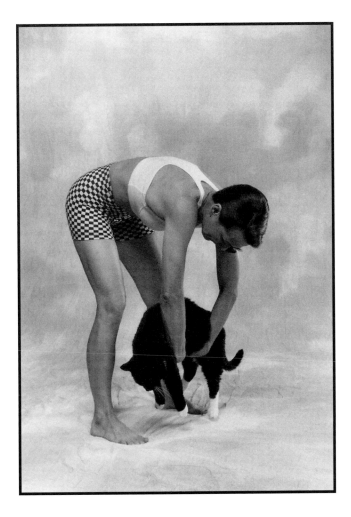

BACK

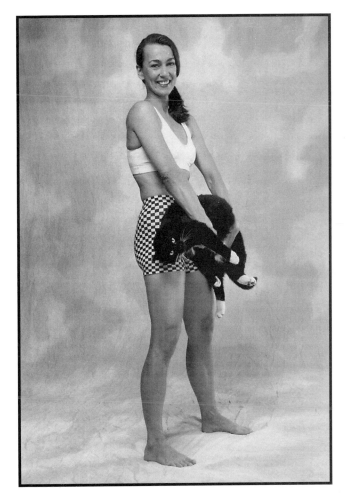

ABDOMINALS

Cat Crunches

Lie on your back with your knees bent at a 90 degree angle. Pick up your cat and raise it directly above your shoulders. With small pressing movements, lift your shoulders toward the ceiling. Keep in mind that the movement is straight up and not toward the knees. Exhale on the lift, inhale when you're coming back down. Don't hold your breath during this exercise and remember to keep your stomach muscles tight. I recommend 3 sets of 20 or as many as you can do.

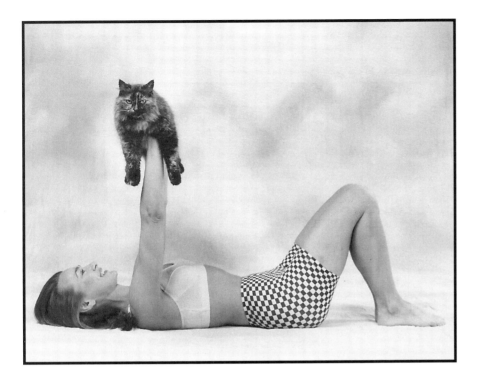

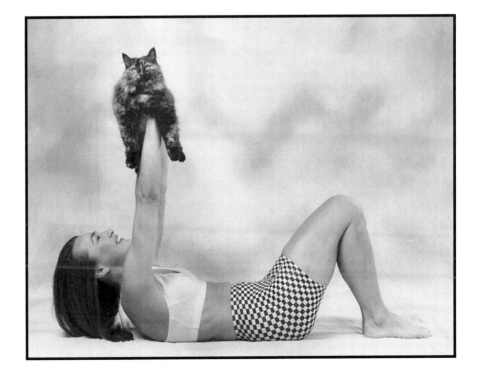

Seated Cat Leg Raise

Sit on the edge of a chair and place your cat snuggly around your ankles. Hold on to the seat and lean back enough so that you have comfortable leverage. Contract your stomach muscles and slowly raise your legs, then slowly lower them. Your cat may slide up and down your legs, which is fine. You don't have to lift your legs high for this exercise to be effective. This is especially good for the lower abdominal muscles. I recommend 3 sets of 12 repetitions.

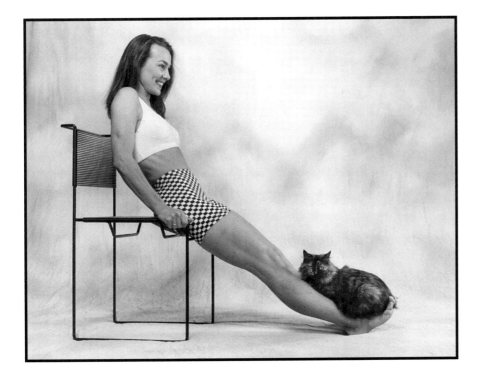

ABS

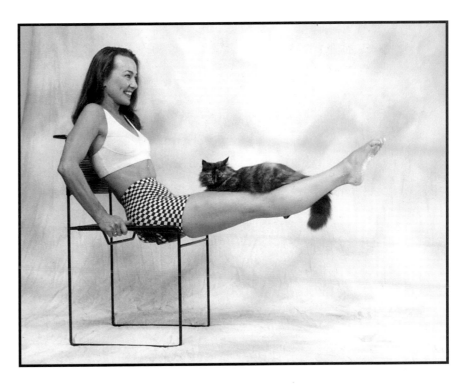

Cat Twists

Stand with your cat across your shoulders and plant your feet shoulder-width apart. Slowly twist your torso and shoulders as far as you can go to the right and return to the starting position. Do not twist your hips, only twist your torso and shoulders! This exercise is great for those "love handles" we end up with at one point or another. Do these slowly and remember to breathe! Do 2 sets of 15 repetitions on both sides.

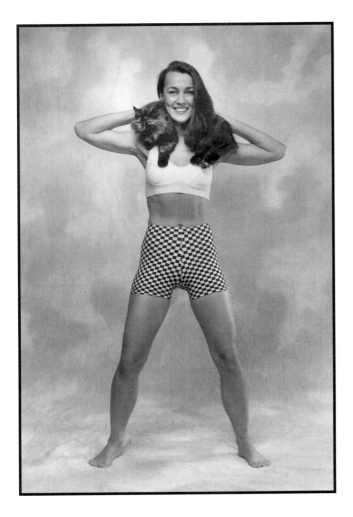

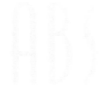

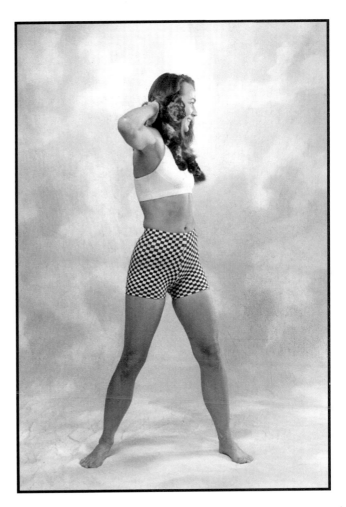

SHOULDERS

Forward Cat Shoulder Raises

Stand with your knees slightly bent and your pelvis gently tucked forward. Don't arch your back. Hold your cat between its front and back legs in a palms-up grip. With your arms extended directly in front of you, exhale as you slowly raise your cat. Do not raise your cat higher than the level of your forehead. Inhale as you slowly lower your cat to the starting position, at shoulder height. Don't let your arms fall below shoulder height and try to keep your neck muscles relaxed during this exercise. I recommend 3 sets of 12 repetitions or less, depending upon the weight of your cat. If this exercise is too difficult or puts strain on your back, you can vary it by holding your cat with your arms in a fully extended position down at your thighs, then raising the cat, using straight arms, to shoulder height.

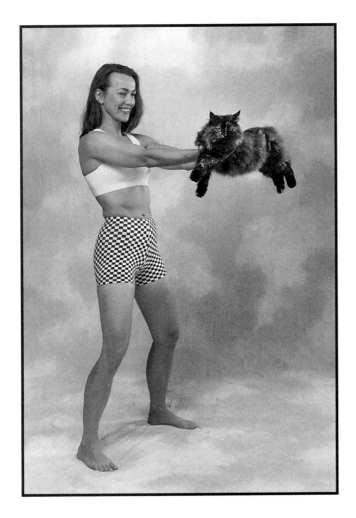

SHOULDERS

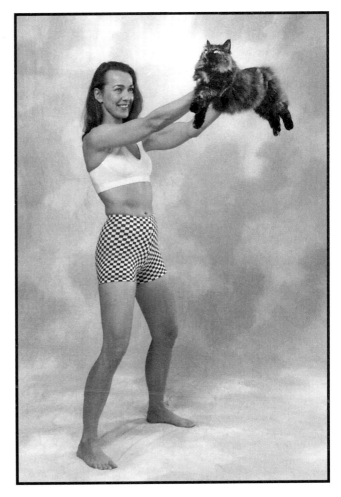

Overhead Cat Press

Stand with your knees slightly bent and hips slightly forward. Hold your cat between its back and front legs and place it gently behind your neck. Bend your head forward slightly and exhale as you raise your cat above your head. Keep your elbows out to the side, and inhale as you lower your cat to your shoulders. Do 3 sets of 12 repetitions.

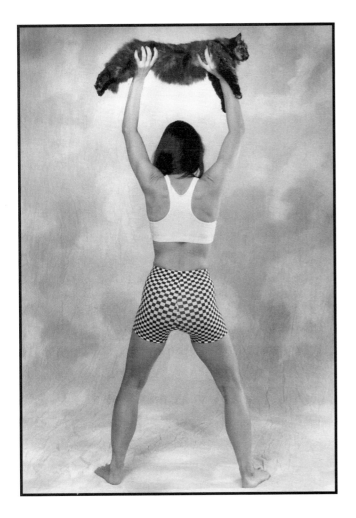

SHOULDERS

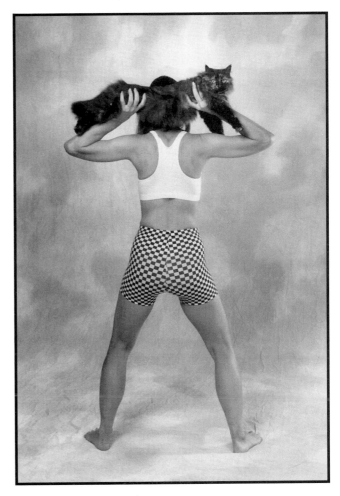

Cat Shrug

Hold your cat using a palms-up grip, with your arms extended to your thighs. Keeping your back straight, and with your feet flat on the ground, pull your shoulders up toward your ears and hold that position for a moment. Relax to starting position. Don't bend your elbows; the only movement here is your shoulders. Breathe normally throughout the exercise. I recommend 3 sets of 12 repetitions.

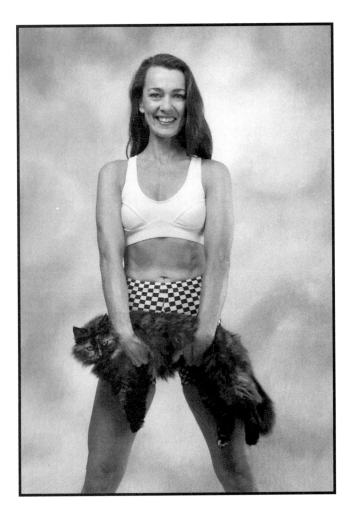

SHOULDERS

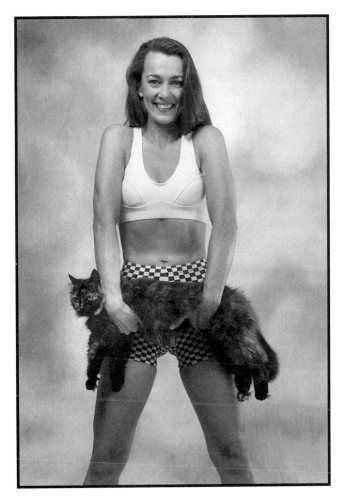

QUADRICEPS AND BUTTOCKS

Cat Squats

Stand erect with your cat across your shoulders. If you or your cat are uncomfortable, place a towel under your cat. Your foot spacing should be a little wider than shoulder width. With your chest held high and your back flat, lower slowly, bending at the knee, until the tops of your thighs are parallel to the floor. Push right back up to starting position. Never round your back and don't attempt to use a heavy cat until you master this technique. Inhale as you descend, exhale as you come up. I recommend 2 sets of 12 repetitions.

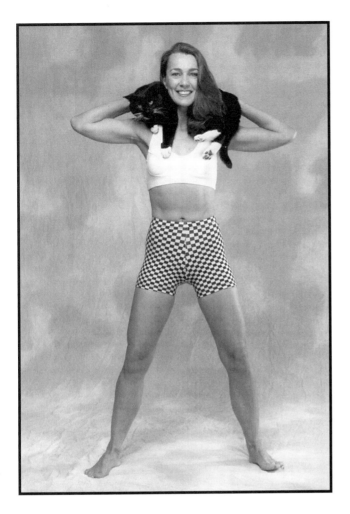

QUADRICEPS &
BUTTOCKS

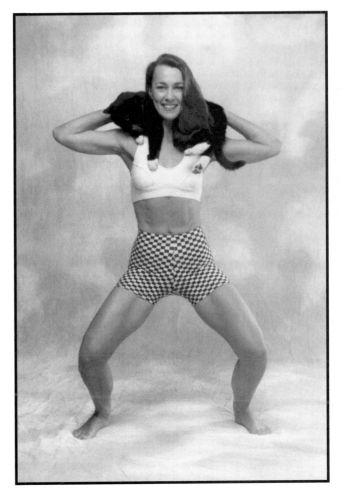

Cat Lunges

Stand erect with your cat across your shoulders. Again, if you are uncomfortable, place a towel under your cat. Take a large step forward, taking care not to let your forward knee move beyond your toe. Inhale, and slowly lower yourself to a squat position, keeping your back leg straight. Exhale, and push off the front leg to return to the standing position. Keep in mind that this exercise is a two-part move. The first part is the large step forward, the second is the downward squat. People often lunge forward, but the lunge is actually the downward motion, when your thigh is horizontal to the floor. Do 3 sets of 12 repetitions on the right leg, and then repeat with the left leg.

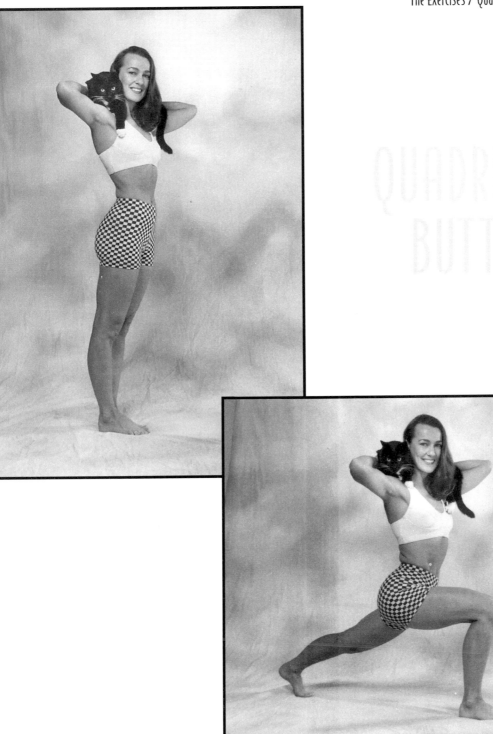

QUADRICEPS &
BUTTOCKS

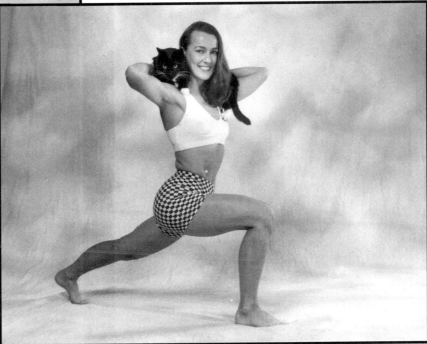

CALVES

Seated Big Cat Calf Raises

Sit in a chair with your feet flat on the ground and place your cat across your lap. Make sure your cat's weight is evenly distributed across both of your legs. Raise up on your toes as high as possible, pausing for a second, and then very slowly return to a relaxed position. I like to use Masi for this exercise because he weighs a ton and I get better resistance. Breathe normally throughout the exercise. I recommend doing 3 sets with 15 repetitions.

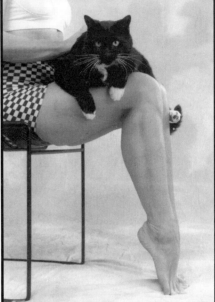

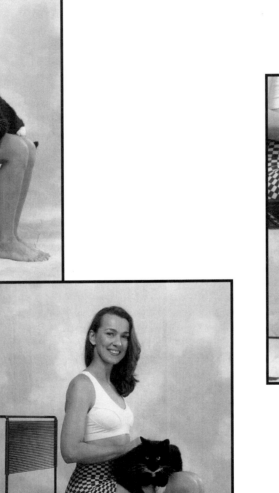

CALVES

Standing Big Cat Calf Raises

You can either place your cat around your shoulders or hold it against your chest for this exercise. Stand on the edge of a step and slowly rise to your toes, flexing your calf muscles. Hold. A railing or a wall to hold on to is ideal to steady yourself. Gently lower yourself until you feel a good stretch. Breathe normally. I recommend 3 sets of 15 repetitions.

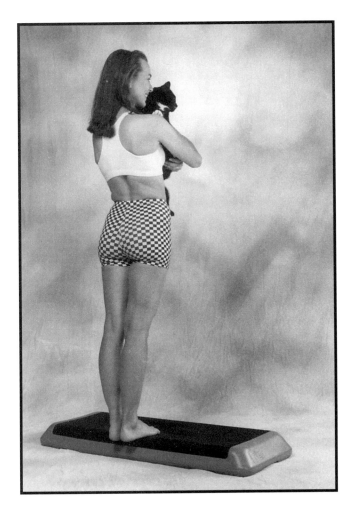

CALVES

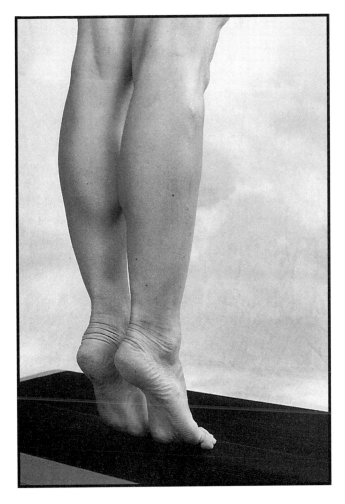

Aerobics and Stretching

NOW YOU'RE HOOKED ON CATFLEXING and so is your cat, and you think it's the greatest thing since sliced bread. You're able to hang out at home with your best buddy and strengthen and tone your muscles. You're starting to look and feel better. What more could you want? YOU CAN'T STOP THERE! Total fitness includes a good weight training program, aerobics, and nutrition. Technically speaking, an aerobic activity is one that increases your heat rate 60 to 80 percent and lasts for at least 20 minutes. To be honest with you, I've had many a night when Bad and I went to town sweating up a storm because we didn't want to rest between our sets. Yes, this would be considered aerobic, however, these times are very few and far between (not to mention that I don't recommend it). Keep in mind that doing any weight training activity fast could result in injury. Now, what are you going to do for your heart and lungs? And how do you think you're going to burn that overall fat? You've got it. Aerobics.

AEROBICS

Because I enjoy music so much, my favorite aerobics activity is dancing, but I also like running, ice skating, rollerblading, and hiking. As I mentioned earlier, I like to warm up with some form of aerobic activity before I begin my Catflexing program, but this is not required. Just getting started on some form of activity is what's important. Simply try to enjoy the exercise and how invigorated it makes your body feel. Once you begin doing it with some regularity and watch your body become even more toned, you'll wonder how you made it this far without it.

Choosing an aerobic activity is simple: Do something you enjoy. Most of you are probably saying, "But I don't know any aerobics." I understand. I know it's tough even thinking about running around after a long day at work, but once you begin, you'll feel rejuvenated.

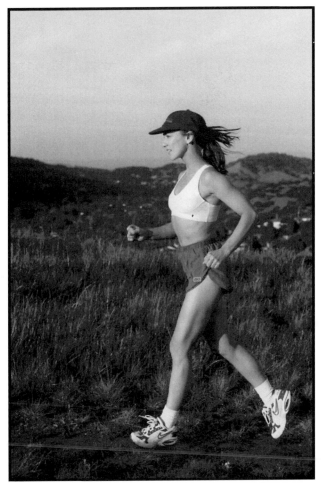

Whatever form of aerobics you choose, you need to do it at least three times a week. Vary your aerobic activities; nothing is set in stone. Try going out dancing or put on some of your favorite music and dance around your house. How about rowing on your favorite lake? What is most important is that you do it with some vigor to get your pulse rate up and that you do it for at least 15 to 20 minutes. You can increase the length of time eventually, but for starters, 15 to 20 minutes is fine.

Here are some popular aerobic activities you can choose from:

Aerobics Classes	Ice Skating
Bicycling	Jumping Rope
Brisk Walking	Rollerblading
Cross-Country Skiing	Rowing
Dancing	Running
Golfing	Stair Climbing
Hiking	Swimming
Hill Climbing	Tennis

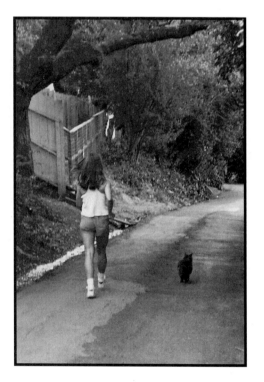

Aerobic activity is just as important for our furry friends. I always recommend spending a good 15 to 20 minutes every other day doing aerobics with your cats. There are many ways to do it. Here are a few ideas to get you started. These are just a few of my suggestions; I'm sure you have your own. Simple combinations of activity and attention for a few minutes here and there can only enhance your pet's optimum level of fitness as well as your closeness to it.

1. Walking. Bad and I have always enjoyed walking together. We walk to the corner and then sprint home. My neighbor also takes her cat for a walk. Some cats really enjoy this, but you'll never know until you try it. I do not recommend this for people who live in busy urban areas.

2. Trailing yarn. Trailing a piece of string or yarn behind you is a game no cat will refuse to play.

3. Retrieval. Whether it's your pet's favorite toy, or a wadded up piece of paper or aluminum foil, some cats get very excited when something is thrown. Masi and I play soccer, in which he's the goalie. I open a shopping bag and place it on the floor. He takes his position directly in front of the bag. I crumble up 10 to 15 pieces of paper and try my best to dart them into the bag. It's very impressive to see how good he's become as he vigorously bats each piece of paper into the air. Perhaps a pro team will pick him up.

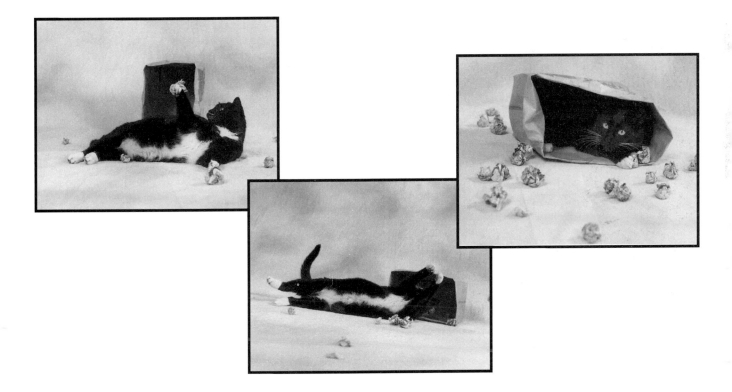

4. Monkey-in-the-middle. Using crumpled paper, or better yet, a fake mouse, you and a friend sit at opposite sides of a room. Toss the mouse in the air or scoot it along the floor while your cat sits in the middle attempting to catch it.

5. Go to your local pet store and see what types of games they have for your cat. I recently purchased a toy called Cat Track. Masi loves it. A ball is housed inside a plastic circular track with spacing enough for your cat's paw to bat the ball but not enough space to remove it, although your cat will go into a tizzy trying. I sometimes think cat toys have been developed for human entertainment.

SSTTRREETTCCHHIINNGG

Stretching is an essential part of an exercise program. The benefits of stretching are numerous, but some of the more important ones are that it allows your muscles to become more elastic which increases your flexibility; it reduces risk of muscle and joint injury and muscle soreness; it helps reduce back strain because the spine is more flexible; and it relaxes muscles, which eases the effects of stress and tension. An added benefit is that, with increased flexibility, you move, look, and feel better.

As for our devoted workout partners, this is the easy part. We don't even have to teach them how to stretch, in fact, we could probably learn something from them. Cats naturally stretch when they clean themselves, and believe me, after a hearty workout, your cat will always want to take a bath. Immediately following our workout, I stretch, and Bad bathes. It's perfect.

The next time your cat bathes, notice how incredibly flexible it is. Cats even use proper technique, holding their positions for long periods of time without bouncing. You'd think they'd taken advanced yoga or something.

There are several different ways to stretch, but the safest technique is the static stretch. This stretch involves holding the stretch in its farthest position, without bouncing, for 5 to 10 seconds, then gently releasing. Becoming flexible takes time, so be easy in your approach. Never force a stretch, and don't hold your breath while stretching—your muscles need the oxygen. The more you stretch, the more flexible you will become.

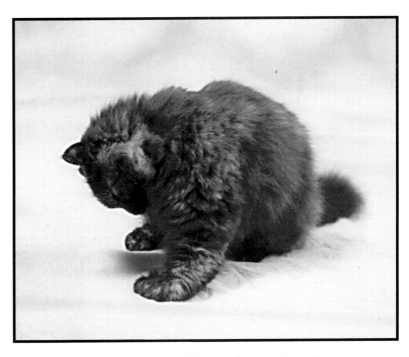

In the following pages, I will show you some basic stretches. Try to hold each stretch for 5 to 10 seconds, relax, then repeat the stretch a couple of times. Stretching should be relaxing, so enjoy yourself! When you become more comfortable with stretching, you can incorporate additional stretches, if you like. Please note: You should not feel any pain. If you do, you are either doing the stretch wrong, or you are overstretching. Some slight discomfort may be expected, but if you feel pain, immediately stop the stretch. You should never feel any extreme pain while stretching.

Leg Crossover Stretch

Stand with one leg crossed in front of the other. Keeping your knees locked, bend over and place your hands on your thighs just above your knees (for the advanced Catflexer, extend your hands to the floor). When you begin to feel the stretch in the back of your legs, stay in that position for 5 to 10 seconds, then gently release and repeat the stretch with the other leg.

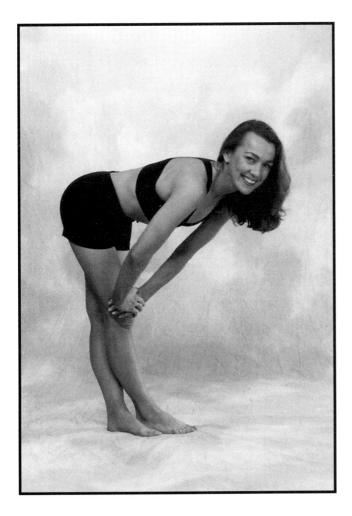

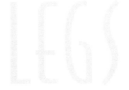

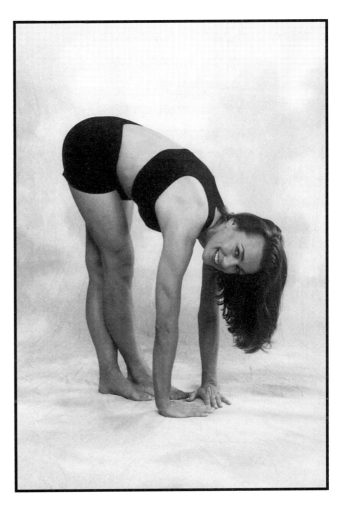

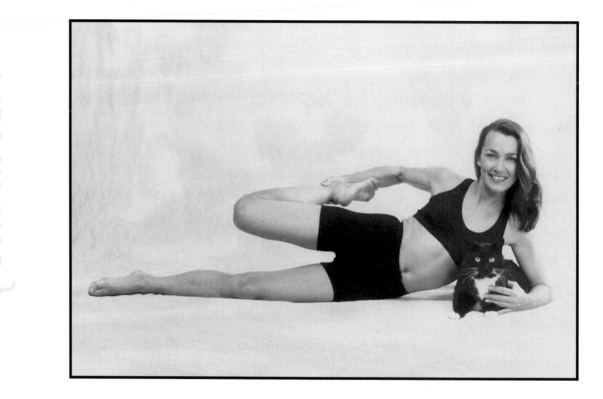

Quadriceps

Lie on your side with your legs together. Bend the upper leg and take hold of your foot, gently pulling it toward your buttocks. When you feel the stretch in the front of your thighs, hold the position for approximately 10 seconds. Turn over and repeat on the other side. If you prefer, you can do this exercise lying on your stomach.

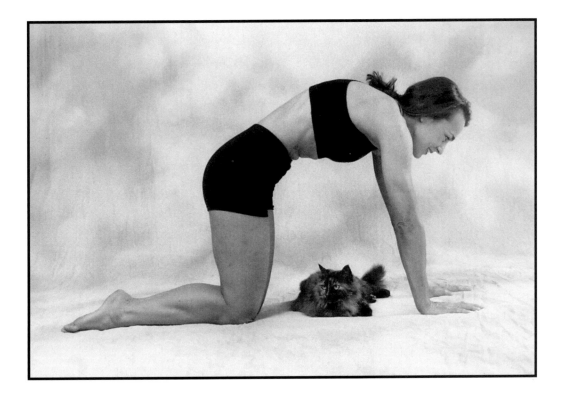

Back

Get down on the floor on your hands and knees and with your knees together. Round your back, arching like a cat. Keep your abdominal muscles tight as you contract to the farthest point possible. Hold the stretch for 5 to 10 seconds, then release, returning to a flat back. Repeat a few more times.

Buttocks and Hips

Lie on your back with your arms extended to the side. Bend both legs and bring your knees up to your chest. Slowly lower both legs to the right, keeping your arms, head, and shoulders flat on the floor. Hold this stretch for 10 seconds. Gently roll your legs to the other side and hold the stretch for 10 seconds. Repeat a few times on both sides.

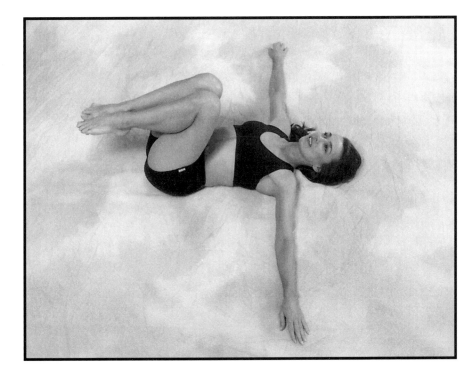

BUTTOCKS & HIPS

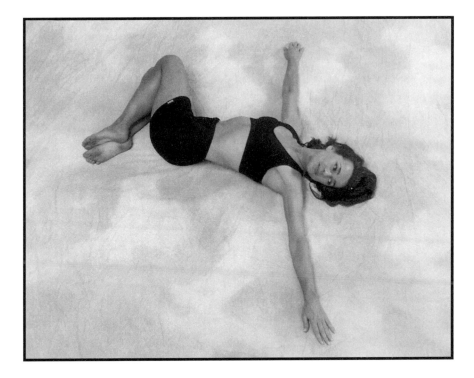

Neck

While standing or sitting, place your hands behind your head, near the crown. Gently pull your head down, tucking your chin into your chest. Hold the stretch, then release. Repeat a few times.

Next, while standing or sitting, place your right hand on the left side of your head, just above your ear. Slowly and gently pull your head toward your right shoulder. When you feel the stretch, hold the position for 5 to 10 seconds, then release. Do the same stretch for the other side. Repeat a few times.

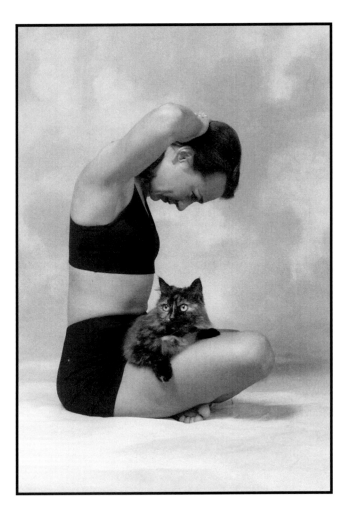

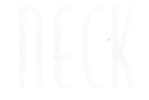

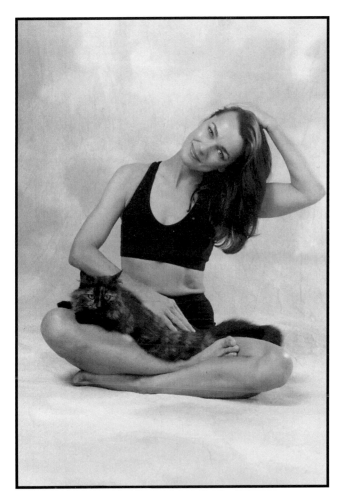

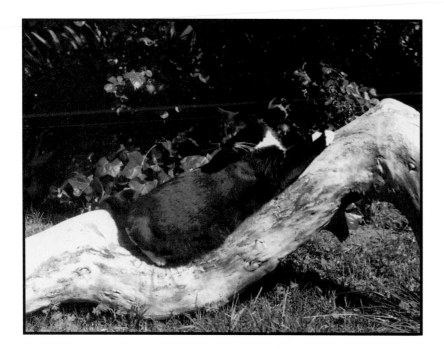

Here's Masi in two of his favorite stretches.

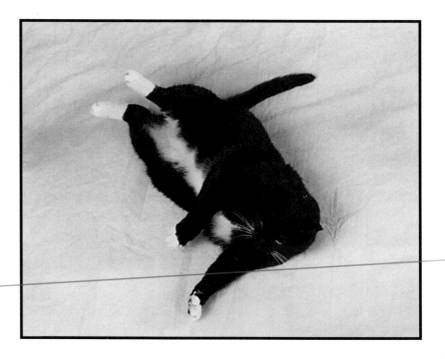

Nutrition

I'VE NEVER HAD A WEIGHT PROBLEM. That doesn't mean I haven't had to pay attention to what I put in my body. Like most people, I get cravings for "bad" food. (I hate to use my cat's name in vain!) When I do, I generally give in. After all, I'm only human, and I can only say no to bonbons for so long. As my nutritional awareness has developed over the years, these cravings have diminished considerably.

Ever since the gut-wrenching war surplus Spam frenzy of the Fifties, there has been an ongoing flux in the nutrition industry. Only in recent years has so much attention been placed on the relationship between exercise and nutrition. Unfortunately, the ideal dietary balance has yet to be established. Who do we listen to? It is understandable how someone could get discouraged. Don't get me wrong, I realize there are diet books that are well researched and diet plans that have helped millions. But think about what the word "diet" implies. To me, it implies restriction, that I must *give up* something. The thought of restriction makes my skin crawl. I know I'm not the only person who feels this way: Of the millions of Americans who go on diets, only about two percent lose weight. So what does that tell you? Dieting alone doesn't work!

Although the concept of dieting is well intended, there is something critical missing—emphasis on a healthy lifestyle. A healthy lifestyle is one in which we revere our bodies, making conscious decisions to do only what is best for it. This includes changing our eating habits and choosing nutritious foods. And exercise, of course, is essential.

People often ask me how I stay so slender as if there is some mystery to it. Believe me, I don't have a body like this by just sitting around eating fluffer-nutter and potato chip sandwiches, and I also don't starve myself. The worst thing you can do for your body is to starve it. If your intention is to lose weight by not eating, it will only be counterproductive. When you starve your body, it instinctively goes into survival mode and protects its fat storage. We will NOT burn fat and our metabolisms slow down. So remember this when you think you should forego your lunch or dinner. I always eat three healthy meals a day and of course exercise regularly...that is a sure way to lose weight. Healthy meals do not consist of foods high in fat and sugar. If you crave foods that promote weight gain, don't feel guilty and beat yourself up too much. It is just as easy to crave healthy food as it is junk food. A little education and time is all that is necessary!

Here are some basic guidelines I follow:

1. Keep fat intake low.

2. Eat complex carbohydrates.

3. Eat food high in fiber.

4. Eliminate refined sugars.

5. Eat adequate protein.

6. Drink at least eight glasses of water each day.

7. Keep your sodium intake low.

FAT

There is nothing wrong with fat. In fact, we need some fat in our diets. There is, however, something wrong with consuming too much fat. When you eat fat, you store fat. Fat is already in its final form, meaning that ice cream cone you ate last night goes directly to your hips! What the statistics say is true: Over 1.5 million Americans will have heart attacks this year; heart attacks are the leading cause of death in the United States. Overconsumption of fat is also linked to heart disease, breast cancer, diabetes, and prostrate and colon cancer. Of the calories consumed by Americans daily, approximately 40 percent are from fat, which means we are eating way above the recommended 15 to 25 grams a day.

On the plus side, fat provides us with energy. It also acts as padding to protect our internal organs. If there is not enough fat in our bodies it becomes difficult for fat-soluble vitamins to be absorbed. But, as average Americans, we don't have to worry about getting enough fat since we eat three to four times the daily requirement already.

The bad guy is saturated fat. Anything oily that remains solid at room temperature is something you want to run from. Saturated fat, which is found primarily in animal and dairy products, is loaded with cholesterol. Cholesterol, at high levels, clogs arteries, which can cause arteriosclerosis and even heart attacks. Cocoa butter and tropical oils such as coconut, palm, and palm kernel are also high in saturated fat and should be avoided. Turn the page for a partial list of foods high in saturated fats—and study up!

Now don't think that just because you can easily eliminate these products all your worries are over. There are two other fats, monounsaturated and polyunsaturated, to look out for. These fats are liquid at room temperature and are mainly found in vegetable and nut oils and fish. We must

FOODS HIGH IN SATURATED FATS

Beef	Ice Cream
Beef Tallow	Ice Milk
Boston Brown Beans	Lamb
Butter	Luncheon Meats
Cake	Milk (Whole, 2%, 1%)
Cheese	Milkshakes
Cheesecake	Non-Dairy Creamers
Chili con Carne	Pompano
Chocolate	Popcorn (microwave)
Cocoa Butter	Pork (bacon, sausage)
Cottage Cheese (4%)	Pudding
Cream	Pumpkin (canned)
Cream- or Butter-Based Sauces	Quiche
Eggnog	Seaweed
Fried Foods (saturated oils)	Soups (cream-based)
Garlic Spread	Turkey (dark meat)
Granola	Tropical Oils
Gravy (brown, packaged)	Veal (fattier cuts)
Hot Dogs	

watch out for these other sneaky fats because both can be hydrogenated. Hydrogenation is a process by which hydrogen is added to monounsaturated or polyunsaturated fat to make it solid. This means they are no longer unsaturated but saturated fats. On the following page is a list of foods that have polyunsaturated fats in them.

So are there *any* fats which are good for you? Earlier, I stated that we need some fat in our diets for energy and for insulation, among other things. Believe it or not, there is such a thing as a "good" fat! Fish oil and flax seed oil both contain Omega-3 and Omega-6 essential fatty acids, which are known to be good sources of nutrition. The good news for athletes is that these oils have also been shown to substantially increase stamina and improve recovery time. Flax seed oil in particular tastes great on salads or vegetables, eaten with bread, or sprinkled on baked potatoes (instead of butter). It should not be heated for cooking. Your local health food store is the best place to find out more about this miracle oil.

Many nutritionists believe that 20 to 30 percent of your total daily caloric intake should come from fat. I feel 15 to 20 percent is better. They also recommend eating no more than 20 to 25 grams of fat a day with little of that being saturated fat. What does all this mean? It means you better start reading your labels and reconsider eating fast foods or snacking on cheese. For instance, fast food hamburgers contain an average of 30 grams of fat per burger. Cheese has an average of 7 to 8 grams of fat per slice. How many times have you stood at the buffet table at a party shoveling in the cheese cubes while you're mustering up the courage to speak with that potential special someone across the room? Or simply leaning on your refrigerator door munching slice after slice while you decide what's for dinner? There are books that list the fat content of each and every food. It's a scary proposition, but I recommend reading them.

FOODS WITH POLYUNSATURATED FATS

Bagels	Lentils	Soybeans
Barbecue Sauce	Nuts	Sweet Potatoes
*Bread	*Popcorn	Tofu
*Corn Chips	*Potato Chips	Vegetable and Nut Oils
Cornmeal	*Salad Dressing	
Fish	Seeds	

FOODS WITH MONOSATURATED FATS

Almonds	Croissants	*Pies
Animal Fats	*Donuts	Pork
Avocados	Eggs	Sausage
*Biscuits	Lard	
*Bread	*Margarine	*Shortening
*Brownies	*Muffins	Veal
*Cake	Oatmeal	
*Cookies	*Peanut Butter	

*often contains hydrogenated oil

Here are a few fast foods fat statistics to get you started. Remember, we're trying to stay in the range of 15 to 25 fat grams per day. Good luck!

PRODUCT	FAT (GRAMS)	CALORIES	% OF CALORIES FROM FAT
Burger King			
Bacon Double Cheeseburger	31	515	54
Croissantwich with Sausage	40	538	68
Double Cheeseburger	27	483	50
Hamburger Deluxe	20	344	50
Jack in the Box			
Bacon Cheeseburger	45	705	57
Chef Salad (dry)	18	325	50
with Thousand Island dressing	48	137	40
Chicken Filet	19	430	38
Kentucky Fried Chicken			
KFC Extra-Tasty Crispy Chicken			
Center Breast	21	344	55
Thigh	31	415	67
KFC Skinfree Crispy			
Center Breast	17	298	49
Thigh	17	256	60
Colonel's Chicken Sandwich	27	482	50

PRODUCT	FAT (GRAMS)	CALORIES	% OF CALORIES FROM FAT
McDonald's			
Chef Salad (dry)	9	170	48
Big Mac	27	500	47
McChicken	20	415	43
Quarter Pounder	20	410	44
Roy Rogers			
Bar Burger	39	611	57
Bacon Cheeseburger	39	590	60
Cheeseburger	36	563	59
Roast Beef with Cheese	20	424	40
Taco Bell			
Beef Burrito	21	431	44
Burrito Supreme	22	440	45
Chicken Fajita	11	226	40
Taco Salad with Shell	61	905	61
Wendy's			
Bacon Cheeseburger Jr.	25	440	51
Big Classic with Cheese	40	638	49
Chicken Club Sandwich	25	520	43
Fish Filet Sandwich	25	460	4

Notice I didn't include French fries? I didn't want to depress you too quickly. On the average, French fries have 10 to 11 grams of fat per 10 fries. The same goes for potato chips. Now, how many times have you sat down and eaten ten potato chips. I guess now you'll be counting.

Moving on to our beloved sweets, what about those chocolates that we can't seem to go without? After viewing the numbers below, you might change your mind.

PRODUCT	FAT (GRAMS)	CALORIES
Almond Joy	14	250
Mounds	14	260
Reese's Peanut Butter Cups (2 cups)	17	280
Snickers (2 oz.)	14	280
Twix	14	280

PRODUCT	FAT (GRAMS)	CALORIES
Caesar	7	70
French	6	60
Italian	7	60
Ranch	6 to 7	60
Roquefort	8	77
Thousand Island	5 to 6	60

So, when you're at the movie theater and want a candy bar, go for the popcorn instead...that is, of course, if it's air popped with no butter added.

Are we ready for salad dressings? And you thought that just because you ate salads you could lose weight. Vegetables alone have no fat. It's the dressing that adds calories. When looking at the above chart, keep in mind that these numbers have been calculated using a SINGLE TABLESPOON of dressing. Yes, you read it right. What I want to know is how many people use only a single tablespoon of dressing on their salads?

What do you think now after looking over these statistics? Are you ready for a lifestyle change yet?

So, now you're in the supermarket armed with all this new knowledge. Good luck! As you well know, everything is labeled fat-free, sugar-free, sodium-free. I always say taste-free, too. Don't buy into this unless you have thoroughly read your labels; even then you could still be fooled. When something says sugar-free, be wary, because it may be loaded with fat. And when the labels say fat-free, check for sugar, which interferes with our fat-burning process. Glittery product labeling makes me leery. If a bag of potato chips says "cholesterol-free" then the product better not have any fat in it because our livers transform fat into cholesterol. If a box of butter cookies says "hydrogenated," then the manufacturer has tricked us again. We have to be scientists just to go grocery shopping. Doesn't all this manipulation get your goat? It's a raw deal. Read your labels; know what you're putting into your body. I can't emphasize this enough.

CARBOHYDRATES

Do you ever feel spaced out or feel like you have no energy to do anything? In all probability you are lacking carbohydrates. Carbohydrates are responsible for your brain power as well as energy for your body to function. "Carbs," popularly known as energy food, are a combination of sugars. These sugars fall into two categories: Simple and complex. The simple carbohydrates are refined sugar and fruit. Like everything else, there are good ones, and not so good ones. (Notice I didn't say "bad.") The carbs we need most in our diets, about 55 to 60 percent, are the complex carbohydrates.

Let's look first at the simple carbohydrates. These are the refined sugar found in cakes and candies, and they have no nutritional value. No matter what anyone tells you, sugar is terrible if you are trying to lose weight. The simple truth is that sugar tricks our metabolism and alters our fat-burning process. Not only that, sugar rots our teeth. Even if you're not trying to lose weight, you're better off avoiding it. Fruit is a simple carbohydrate, but it's unrefined and is extremely high in nutritional value. Fruit is the better choice when you have a hankering for sweets.

Complex carbohydrates provide us with long-lasting energy; they also give a satiated feeling which curbs our appetite for fats and sweets. Complex carbohydrates are high in fiber which, studies reveal, is excellent for our colons. Carbohydrates high in fiber include vegetables, pasta, rice, whole grains, and cereals. When choosing grains, try to choose whole grains, brown breads such as whole grain or wheat, pastas, and rice. Include fibers from different sources in your daily diet and choose only high-fiber cereals without added sweeteners.

PROTEIN

The recommended amount of daily protein is two or three servings of approximately 3 ounces each. That is not a lot! Have you ever gone to a nutritionist or doctor who recommended you actually eat that 18 to 21 ounce T-bone steak? Many people think that protein is the most important element of a healthy diet and therefore it should be the largest percentage of our daily diet. Protein is very important, but what is most important is a balance between all the food groups.

Bodybuilders and Catflexers wouldn't be able to develop muscles without protein because it is the main building block for our bodies. So if you are a weight trainer and a Catflexing enthusiast, then you will need a little more than the recommended 15 percent. Protein is also responsible for the maintenance of our hair, nails, skin, blood vessels, and internal organs. It affects our hormone production, which controls our growth, metabolism, and sexual development. Fat is often found in protein sources, so when selecting them, consider skinless chicken, low-fat fish, egg whites, beans, and nonfat yogurt, milk, and cottage cheese. Choose only lean meat, and trim all noticeable fat. If you are a vegetarian, some good protein sources are egg whites, white cheeses, skim milk, cottage cheese, beans, lentils, potatoes, and corn.

REFINED SUGAR

We don't have to be brain surgeons to understand that anything stripped of its nutritional value can't be good for us. Refined sugar, and what it does to the metabolism, is often the culprit behind weight gain. Consuming sugar releases glucose in the bloodstream, and when too much glucose is released, it causes insulin to be produced. When we produce insulin, we lose the enzyme responsible for removing fat from fat cells. So only in small, occasional doses, please.

LOWER YOUR SODIUM INTAKE

I don't know about you, but I'm one of those people who is very sodium sensitive. When I eat too much salt, my body swells, I feel like I've gained twenty pounds, and the next day I feel like Linda Blair in *The Exorcist*. My cats don't even want to get near me.

Normal sodium levels range from 1,500 to 2,400 milligrams a day. Unless you are advised by your doctor to reduce your levels or you have a sensitivity to salt, you should try to maintain this recommended allowance. After all, sodium is important to our system as it regulates our body fluids. Salt is also important when we take on an exercise program because it allows our muscles to contract.

DRINK LOTS OF WATER

Water flushes the excess salt and toxins from our bodies and helps to eliminate the fat from our systems. Most people don't know that drinking lots of water prevents water retention and curbs our appetites. Water also keeps our skin looking moist and refreshed. I think water is the cure-all. If you feel toxic, bloated, fat, hungry between meals, or look in the mirror and see something like a shar-pei, I advise drinking a glass of water.

I always recommend drinking a couple of glasses of water before working out and then every 20 to 30 minutes into the workout. Sometimes we don't realize the amount of moisture we lose. Another secret is that water helps give us the energy to work out. Try exercising when your water reserves are low; you'll feel like a lead bolt. You can never get enough water, so drink up!

Cat Nutrition

THE MOST LOVING CHOICE WE CAN MAKE for our furry friends is to select healthy foods for them. Like human nutrition, cat nutrition is an ever-evolving science. A diet consisting of protein, carbohydrates, fats, vitamins, minerals, and water is essential. Sound familiar? Unfortunately, the minimum nutritional requirements have yet to be established, leaving us in a pickle when deciding what is healthiest for our loved ones. Because we can never be sure if our cats' nutritional needs are being met, providing them with a diverse diet is essential.

Here's a quiz to test your knowledge of cat nutrition. Answers are true or false.

1. By-products are healthy for your cat.

2. Ethoxyquin is an important mineral in many cat foods.

3. Dogs need twice the amount of B vitamins in their diets as cats.

4. A high-fat diet is fine for cats, and we're talking saturated fats, the kind doctors tell us to stay away from.

5. Cats by nature are not finicky.

6. For cats, variety is the spice of life.

7. Ham and pork can clog your cat's blood vessels.

8. When purchasing cat food, make sure taurine is one of the ingredients.

9. There is no such thing as a healthy vegetarian cat.

How did you do? Should I give you the answers? Alright. Read on.

What this means is simply to supplement your cat's diet with food from various sources, especially protein sources. Wild, or feral, cats have always chosen foods from different sources—birds, small rodents, frogs, toads, insects. Another reason to provide variety is each cat has individual dietary requirements.

Every pet food company has its own set of ingredients, vitamins, and minerals. For instance, one food may be low in vitamin A, while another may be low in the B vitamins but have ample vitamin A. Our pets may not show symptoms of any dietary deficiencies, but once the damage is done it's hard to reverse.

Providing our pets with only one food source is one way to set them up for nutritional deficiencies. Indulging food preferences is another. Just because your cats might like the taste of antifreeze, you wouldn't feed it to them, would you? I realize, as parents, we want to please our pets. However, catering to their every whim is a guarantee for future health problems. Cats then either refuse or become very hesitant to try new foods because they know that if they wait it out, they will get what they want. It's not that cats are finicky, they are just extremely smart! We, the parents, produce picky eaters! Contrary to popular belief, cats are not naturally finicky.

I try to provide my cats with a diet that will enable them to live long and healthy lives. My cats rely on me for their daily food, and I rely on the pet food companies. Unfortunately, there are some commercial pet food companies, more than I would like to admit, that provide our cats with substandard ingredients and use more preservatives and additives than actual food.

Mind you, though, they have great-looking labels and huge names behind them. It is important to read the labels and purchase your pet's food from a pet food store, not a grocery store—unless, of course, this grocery store has high-quality pet foods. Reading labels, though, won't help if you don't know what you're looking for.

What ingredients should you look for? Shop for foods that use the most natural, whole ingredients from each of the five major food groups, avoiding by-products and processed grains. When evaluating ingredients, think of only those foods you would eat yourself as acceptable. I know there is no redeeming value in chicken beaks and toenails (known as by-products). Who, in their right mind, would eat such things? The lesson here is what's good for the goose is good for the gander.

Also, avoid products with artificial flavors and colors, preservatives, or dyes. These chemical additives sabotage the feline's natural state. They have been found to be the cause of many of our cats' health problems, especially allergic reactions.

These are just a few chemicals frequently found in our cat food:

- **Ammoniated glycyrrhizin,** licorice, is known to cause headaches, muscle weakness, and raise blood pressure. It can cause asthma, intestinal upsets, and contact dermatitis.

- **BHA** (butylated hydroxyanisole) is used to preserve fats and oils in foods. It is known to cause allergic reactions and to affect liver and kidney functions. Additional studies are required to determine the safety of current levels used.

- **BHT** (butylated hydroxytoluene) is another preservative for fats and oils. It too can cause allergic reactions. In studies done on pregnant mice, the mice gave birth to offspring that frequently had chemical abnormalities in the brain and subsequent abnormal behavior patterns. BHT is prohibited in

England. The FDA (Federal Department of Agriculture) is pursuing further study of this preservative.

- **Ethoxyquin** is an antioxidant preservative and herbicide, known to cause tumors in mice.

- **Phosphoric acid** is a preservative used to keep products fresh and sweet. It has been known to cause irritations to the skin and mucus membranes.

- **Potassium sorbate** is a preservative known to cause skin irritations.

- **Propyl gallate** is used as an antioxidant. It has been known to cause stomach and skin irritations.

- **Propylene glycol** causes central nervous system depression and kidney changes in some animals.

- **Sodium nitrate,** also called saltpeter, is used as a color fixative. It is known to cause tumors and pancreatic cancer in laboratory animals. It has also been known to cause death by reducing oxygen flow to the brain.

This scary list doesn't even include commonly used dyes, colorings, sugars, salts, artificial flavors, or scents. All of these ingredients are added to stimulate our pet's taste buds. The colorings are added to appease us, the consumer. I recently went to the local grocery store to buy a few boxes of commercial cat food to study their ingredients. Believe me, I never feed my cats this stuff. I brought them home and lined them up on my living room floor. I kept the boxes closed while I compared their ingredients. Then the cats discovered them. Well, you would have thought that a truck full of live mice carrying mackerel were packed in each box. My cats went wild, panting and scratching to get into these boxes. They were high just standing next to them! I was asking myself, what is wrong with this picture? It was only after reading about food additives that I understood why they responded that way. Their reaction validated everything I had read. Many pet food manufacturers add an alarming amount of food additives to cat food to hook cats. Our cats love the product and you, the consumer, buy it for them because you want to please them. Granted, you didn't know any better. Well, now you do!

Research shows that most of the food additives are often the cause of ailments in pets. Animals can be just as sensitive to the foods they ingest as humans, and probably even more so. Here's a good example: My cat Bad had a chronic skin problem. She had, at times, practically eaten her backside raw. I tried everything, including giving her baths and brushing her daily. Initially I thought her condition was a result of fleas. I finally took her to three veterinarians for their recommendations since my home diagnosis had failed. Each of them immediately suggested a cortisone shot. I reluctantly conceded. After the shot, and for the next six weeks, Bad proceeded to sit in the dish cupboard with her head in the corner and her eyes glazed over. The doctor said that some cats are more sensitive than others and have reactions to this drug. When he told me it would last for about six to eight weeks, I nearly clobbered him! I felt awful about making such a poor, uniformed decision and that Bad had to endure such a long and horrible "drug" trip. Time passed and eventually the cortisone wore off. And guess what? Her problem came back. Then it hit me. Could it be dietary? I researched cat nutrition and changed her diet immediately. Bad's new diet included food supplements containing vitamins A and E, fish oils with Omega-3 essential fatty acids, and lecithin. I also changed the hard food she was eating and added various protein sources to her diet such as chicken, lamb, beef, and turkey. After a couple of weeks her problem completely subsided and has yet to come back.

It is imperative that you choose your animal's food wisely and watch for changes in their behavior. And on the next trip you take to the vet, investigate their nutritional awareness. If you're given the deer-in-the-headlights look, I strongly suggest finding another health care provider. I really mean that! Imagine getting a medical check-up and discovering you have high blood pressure, yet your doctor neglects to suggest that you stay away from fats, cholesterol, alcohol, caffeine, and cigarettes. Generally speaking, veterinarians are not nutritionists. Traditional medicine is rooted in a drug-oriented approach. Drugs often treat the symptom and not the cause of an ailment. Although medication is extremely important in helping our animals' medical problems, prevention of these problems through proper diet is grossly overlooked.

Now we get to the fun section: By-products. If you have ever wondered what this means, relax—you're about to find out. I guarantee you're never going to forget either.

Go to the kitchen and take a look at the ingredients on a can or box of commercial cat food. Most of you will find some form of meat by-product or other animal by-product as the first or second ingredient. By-products are meats that comes from the "4 Ds"—dead, dying, diseased, and disabled animals. The federal government actually allows this. According to Dr. P. F. McGargle, a veterinarian and former federal meat inspector, meat by-products can include moldy, rancid, or spoiled processed meats as well as tissue too severely riddled with cancer to be eaten by people. Another veterinarian defined by-products as diseased tissue, pus, hair, assorted slaughterhouse rejects, and carcasses in varying stages of decomposition which are then sterilized with chemicals, heat, and pressure procedures. Doesn't that sound yummy? By the time they process this meat to rid it of all the bacteria and viruses, do you think there are any nutrients left over? I highly doubt it. This brings us back to the additives. It's a vicious cycle. Get the gist? In other words, meat by-products are not healthy for your cat. I hope you didn't get this one wrong on the test.

Now let's get down to the meat and potatoes of the matter. As with humans, cats need protein, carbohydrates, and fats, along with vitamins, minerals, and water for proper development. However, their digestive systems and metabolism are uniquely feline and different from humans. There are many differences in nutritional needs between humans and cats. I'll give you a few of the biggies.

1. Cats have a much higher protein requirement than humans. Cats must have a daily supply of protein. Unlike humans, they are unable to store protein.

2. There is no such thing as a healthy vegetarian cat. Cats have difficulty utilizing vegetable protein.

3. Cats can only absorb vitamin A from animal protein. Humans absorb it from plant sources as well.

4. High-fat diets are not detrimental to cats. They are able to metabolize and digest saturated fats extremely well.

5. Cats need more niacin in their diets than we do because they cannot manufacture it themselves.

6. Cats are extremely sensitive to preservatives.

PROTEINS

Cats are true carnivores and protein is their main building block, aiding in the development and strengthening of muscles. Cats also use protein for energy. (Humans and dogs use carbohydrates for energy.) Remember, cats cannot store excess protein, so it is important they receive a daily supply. Cats need at least 30 percent protein in their daily diet. Sources of protein should only be found in high-quality meats such as beef, turkey, chicken, and lamb. These lean muscle sources are considered to be the most efficient sources of protein, providing the highest ratio of amino acids, vitamins, and minerals. Fish, egg yolk, whole egg, organ meats, whole milk, wheat germ, and corn-meal are also high-quality protein sources. Meat by-products are not considered high-quality sources. Pork and ham should not be fed to your cats either because they have the capacity to clog blood vessels. Pork products contain very large fat globules. Not only that, hot dogs, bacon, and sausages have extremely high levels of preservatives, colorings, and nitrites in them.

Cats also require the proper ratio of essential amino acids, another reason why feeding your cats high-quality proteins as opposed to by-products is crucial. Taurine is one of the essential amino acids. Unfortunately, 80 percent of taurine is lost during the meat cooking process; therefore it must be added. It is an important ingredient to look for when choosing your cat's food. Eggs have a high amount of taurine, but eggs must be cooked before feeding them to your cats because raw egg whites are very difficult for cats to digest. Cats with diets deficient in taurine can develop retinal degeneration and possible blindness, fatal heart muscle disease, immune system dysfunction, blood clotting disorders, and problems related to liver detoxification. Very little taurine is found in dog food, which is one reason why you should never feed your cat dog food. Dog food is generally cereal-based with little taurine, and besides that, cats need twice the amount of protein dogs need.

CARBOHYDRATES

There is no such thing as a healthy vegetarian cat. Cats get their supply of amino acids, vitamins, and minerals from animal proteins, they do not get it from plants. Carbohydrates, therefore, are not essential; however, they generally make up about 20 percent of our cats' diet. Carbohydrates do provide the fiber and bulk needed for intestinal movement. High-quality sources are fruits, vegetables, whole grains, rice, and wheat bran.

FATS

Cats are lucky—a healthy daily diet for them can contain up to 40 percent fat. We're talking about chicken fat, bacon grease, and butter, the soft fats. These fats carry the fat-soluble vitamins A, D, E, and K and supply linoleic acid and arachidonic acid, which are fundamental to the health of your cats. A cat deficient in these essential fatty acids may develop poorly, have dry hair, scaly skin, and be listless and prone to infection. Hard fats, the inferior fats, are more difficult for cats to digest and utilize. The fats they are unable to use will either be stored in the liver or vomited. Cats who eat hard fats are generally fat and greasy. The oils permeate their coats through their glands. Think of what it must do to your couch! Hydrogenated coconut oils should also be avoided because it can cause fatty liver disease.

WATER

Access to clean, fresh water is most important for your pet's health. It is natural for cats to go without food for a long time, but not without water. If they lose up to 10 percent of their moisture, it can be deadly. The amount of water your cat drinks depends on the types of foods it eats as well as temperature, exercise, and illness. Canned foods contain about 75 percent water. This is one of the reasons I never saw my cats drink. They were getting most of their water from the food I was serving. If you never see your cat drink

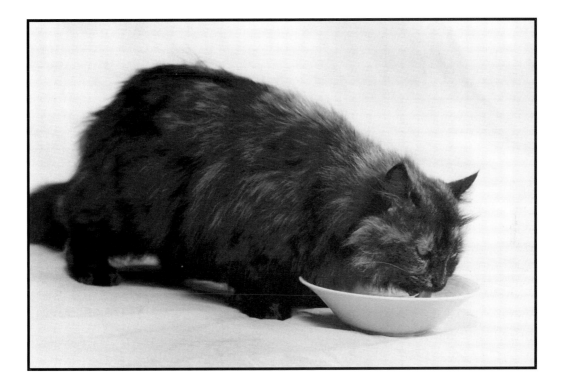

water, don't panic; it's probably related to the food you provide, or they're getting it from a favorite watering hole. Regardless, always provide a clean bowl of water daily.

FREE-FEEDING

Cats in the wild don't have food available to them at all times. Birds don't simply fly up to them and say, "It's time, I'm ready to die, please eat me." In the wild, if they are lucky, cats may eat once a day. Therefore, brief periods of fasting are as natural to them as eating. When cats eat, blood travels to their stomach to aid in the digestive process. During a fast, the blood is available for other functions, such as healing. Fasting also helps keep the intestines, urinary tract, lungs, and pores spic and span. I am not suggesting withholding food for days at a time.

Keeping in synch with what Nature intended is the best approach for the overall health of your cat. Feeding your cat twice a day, mornings and evenings, is the healthiest, most loving method of regulating her diet. Thirty minutes after feeding your cat, remove the food, and, if possible, clean the area. Half an hour gives your cat time to come back to the plate for a second nibble. (Some cats don't eat everything at once.) Keeping the feeding area clean is important: If the area smells like food, irregardless of whether there is food there, the olfactory center of the cat's brain will be stimulated, and the digestion process will be activated.

Here are some more reasons why removing food between meals is important:

1. As I just stated, the smell of food triggers the olfactory center of the cat's brain that tells their body to prepare for digestion. Their metabolisms slow down and blood centers in the stomach, leaving all the other organs undersupplied with blood.

2. The nutritional value of food is diminished when it sits out all day.

3. The risk of feline urologic syndrome (FUS) is greater. Studies have revealed that every time a cat smells food, its urine becomes more alkaline. FUS germs flourish in an alkaline urine.

4. Being involved in your cat's mealtime is important. Preparing your cat's meals, even if it means opening a can of food, builds that special bond between you and your cat.

5. Keeping food out all day is the main cause of the finicky eater syndrome; the constant smell of food short-circuits the hunger reflex.

Try this on your cat after years of free feeding and see if you don't get a reaction. After implementing this change, I discovered that Masi didn't like it one bit. He paced his feeding area all afternoon and then finally came up and bit me on the leg. Now that's gratitude for you. As a parent, I sympathized with him and wanted to give in, but I knew I couldn't. I knew this change would take some time. It was only a couple of days later that he began to adjust. He still lapses in and out, but we're working on a lifestyle change here. That's big. Bad, on the other hand, was always a two-time-a-day eater. She wasn't even fazed by the routine change, but then again, nothing ever fazes her. Some cats naturally eat only twice a day. Other cats, like my fat cat Masi, live near the dish and I now know why. His system was always ready for digestion, therefore, his life centered around food. The last thing you want is a fat, unhealthy cat. Cats do no fare well when they are overweight. They can become sickly and tend to have a slow metabolism.

What if you have an erratic schedule? There is some flexibility here. If you come home at a different hour every day, by all means feed your cat when you get home; a couple of hours will not make a bit of difference. If you are sometimes away for the night, you can leave the food out. Occasional breaks in the routine are okay.

The bottom line? Choose your cat's food wisely, feed him only high-quality sources twice a day, and never overfeed your cat anything but love.

Questions and Answers

Q. I have been Catflexing with my cat Manhattan for approximately two years. I had no idea there so many other Catflexers out there until recently, when I entered my first contest. It was only a local exhibition, but the participation was incredible! Manhattan and I are now preparing for our second contest, but he's acting different this time. He's very irritable and aggressive. My neighbors have told me he's been attacking their cats sexually. What's going on?

A. A change in behavior is always something to be concerned with. Hard training could be the reason for his actions, but I suspect something else is going on. Have you changed his diet? Are his nutritional needs being met? Sometimes cranky behavior is due to a dietary factor. Are you overtraining him to the point where he's upset and angry? You definitely don't want to jeopardize your pet's health. Are you perhaps taking steroids and have left the bottle cap open? Could Manhattan have gotten into them? I suggest taking him to your vet and having a thorough check-up.

Q. I just found out my cat Emmy is pregnant and will be having a litter soon. Is working out in her condition safe?

A. First of all, it's always good to get a veterinarian's approval on the overall condition of your pregnant cat, but generally speaking, cats are a hearty breed. When Bad was pregnant we continued our exercise program almost to the very end! I know it helped me because of her additional weight; rotating your weights is a good practice. Although we took it easy, I know it helped her stay in shape as well. Bad and I actually competed in her later stages of pregnancy. The judges didn't know this, and I think her additional weight helped me look more pumped. We won the contest! She was so excited she went into labor and delivered four kittens in my gym bag!

Q. I'm not very coordinated and I find some Catflexing positions to be very awkward. While doing the Standing Catbell Press, I dropped my cat Booie and she landed on her head. I took her to the emergency vet and they found she had a concussion. She's better now, but she's skittish and reluctant to do the workouts with me. I'm also surprised that she didn't land on her feet. What should I do?

A. One of the reasons Booie landed on her head was that she totally trusted you and was completely caught off guard when you dropped her. Regaining her trust will take some time and patience. I suggest that you don't force the issue. Allow her to come to you. Use your regular handheld weights for now, and do your normal workout in front of her. Pick up Booie intermittently and give her a hug, then put her down and continue with your workout. This shows her that you are not forcing anything on her. When she feels it's time to give it a go again, she'll let you know.

Q. My husband is preparing for a Catflexing competition and is thinking about shaving my cat Kiwi's entire body. I'm furious at the thought, and I'm sure Kiwi would be, too. What would the judges say about this?

A. Good question! I've only seen a few partially shaved cats and most of them were in the hospital for an operation. We will probably be seeing much more of this in the near future. Many professional athletes do it, so why not cats? Personally, I am opposed to it, but I've heard that some cats actually don't mind it, and it's not as traumatic as one would think. The main reason for shaving is to be able to see the muscle definition when competing. Also, when oil is applied, it is much easier to remove it from their skin than it is from their fur. Your cat will have less hairballs, too.

Q. What are the rules about accessories? My cat Evie looks so adorable in her pink collar and pink cat bell. I want her to wear it during competition.

A. There is no ruling at present on accessorizing. To help you decide, think of when Katerina Witt appeared in the 1988 Olympics wearing too much makeup. The judges were surprised. However, her excessive makeup didn't distract them from seeing her true talent. The judges are looking for the overall composition of your routine, the use of proper technique, and a well-trained cat. The judges may not like the look or sound of your cat's bell, but if you and your cat give a thorough performance, that is what they will see.

Q. I have two cats, Norton and Jimmy, but only Norton is interested in Catflexing. I've taken the time to try to integrate Jimmy into my workout programs, but he still doesn't like the unusual handling. My cats have always gotten along, but since I've been Catflexing with Norton, Jimmy has become very jealous and attacks Norton frequently. I want my happy family back. What should I do?

A. There are a couple of things you can do in this situation. First, when you are Catflexing, you must put Jimmy outside or in another room. If you have a toy, give it to him so he is distracted from trying to get out of the room. If you put him outside, I suggest you close your curtains and blinds. Cats are very sneaky and suspicious and don't miss a trick. Second, regardless if it's before or after your Catflexing time, spend some quality time with Jimmy and do some things he likes to do. Put Norton out of the room while you spend this time with Jimmy. Also, talk to Jimmy about what is going on. Your cats understand more than we give them credit for. It's not our actual words they hear; they understand energy, and tone, and they receive the feelings behind what we are trying to say.

Q. I don't have a cat, but I do have a pet macaw named Maxx. Can I flex with him?

A. Many people have asked me about flexing with their pets, from Yorkshire terriers to lizards. The answer is yes if there is mutual interest in working out together. Birds are particularly good at flexing as they play dead and enjoy the swinging motion of some of the flexing moves, and although they don't weigh much, it's better than using no weight at all. When using light weights, I recommend higher repetitions. I was recently asked about using a pet boa for flexing. For those people who like and need heavier weights, boas or other large reptiles are great flexing partners.

Q. My neighbor has been Catflexing for about a year now. At first, when I saw her wielding her Siamese, frankly, I thought she was nuts. Very soon thereafter I witnessed her little Yorkie running around in a frenzy until my friend picked her up and incorporated her into the routine. I've never seen her so close with her pets. I'm jealous. My problem is that I'm terribly allergic to animal fur. I want to Catflex, too. Do you have any suggestions?

A. How unfortunate for you and others with pet allergies. Aside from the obvious, the workout, you miss the incredible bonding that occurs during these sessions. Realistically, I only see two solutions. First, you could see an allergist and go through the testing to identify exactly what gives you an allergic reaction. In most cases, it is not animal fur but the oils on the fur. If this is the case, you may find that some cats don't give you a reaction. Second, I would suggest finding a hairless creature for your companionship. The sphinx would be a perfect breed—it's a cat without hair. However, the sphinx can be extremely expensive and hard to find. You might consider reptiles as an alternative. Snakes and lizards make wonderful pets.

Q. My husband and I both want to Catflex, but we have only one cat. Is it asking too much of our little Sammy to give it a go sometimes twice a day?

A. This may be a lot of stimulation for an animal, but hey, maybe Sammy is one of those exceptional cases. Rely on your pet's feedback. If Sammy wants to do it, go for it! But be careful. The more Sammy exercises, the more food he'll need, and he'll need extra water. Working out twice a day can be dehydrating. If Sammy doesn't want to work out twice daily, rotate your workouts with your pet, and use your handheld weights in between.

Q. I'm an avid Catflexing fan, and I think my cat El is also, but she has one problem. I'm sure you understand—her problem is my problem! During our workout, El passes gas. It happens each and every time. I'm concerned there is something medically wrong. I couldn't take it anymore, so we've stopped Catflexing. I miss our exercise program.

A. I would definitely have her looked over by your vet. It sounds like a simple dietary problem, perhaps lactose intolerance. There is a tablet you can give your cat to reduce gas, just like for humans, but I would talk to your vet before giving it to her.

Q. I have two cats, Brookey and A2. Brookey is a little scrawny cat and A2 is an enormous tom. How do I incorporate their different weights into a solid workout program?

A. Actually, you are very lucky because interchanging weights is very beneficial for muscle development. I suggest that you use Brookey for your toning and definition, and use A2 for building muscle. This is what I do with Bad and Masi. I do an all-around program using Bad because she doesn't weigh much. But when it comes to specific muscles I want to develop more, such as my chest and quads, I always use Masi. Fat cats do come in handy.

If you have any questions or concerns, write to:

Dr. Stefeline Catson
P. O. Box 3598
San Rafael, CA 94912

Animals are very sensitive. They struggle with self-esteem and are often traumatized by neglect. Take time with your pets. Make them feel like a valuable part of the family. Also, please be responsible and spay or neuter your pets. It is a truly loving gesture.

Index

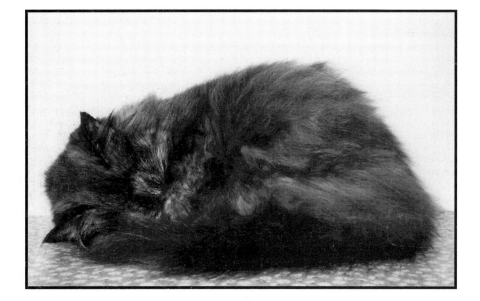